Bey einer Versammlung der Einwohner der Stadt Lancaster, gehalten auf dem Courthaus, Donnerstags, den 19ten September, 1793, um den jezigen beunruhigenden Zustand des bösartigen Fiebers, das in der Stadt Philadelphia graßiret, in Ueberlegung zu nehmen.

Jasper Yeates, Vorsizer.

Ward Beschlossen,

Daß wir es als unsere Pflicht erachten, solche Maasregeln zu ergreifen, die den Endzweck haben zu verhüten, damit das bösartige Fieber welches in der Stadt Philadelphia und andern Orten graßiret, sich nicht in diese Stadt verbreite.

Beschlossen, Daß es denen Kaufleuten und andern Einwohnern anempfohlen werde, sich der Einführung einiger Waaren, sie mögen Namen haben wie sie wollen, in diese Stadt oder deren Nachbarschaft auf vier Wochen lang, zu enthalten. Den Artikel des Salzes von Plätzen die nicht inficirt sind ausgenommen.

Beschlossen, Daß wir die neuliche Empfehlung der Corporation an die hiesigen Besizer der Postwägen, um das Fahren der Postwägen zwischen der Stadt Philadelphia und dieser Stadt einzustellen, damit die Gemüther der Einwohner beruhiget würden, höchstens billigen; und daß wir alles das in unserer Macht stehet anwenden wollen, das Fahren besagter Postwägen und aller anderer Fuhrwerke, so lange die jezige epidemische Seuche dauert, zu verhindern, und daß keine kranke, inficirte Leute in diese Stadt kommen.

Beschlossen, Daß aus jeder Ward acht Personen ernannt werden sollen diese Schlüsse in Vollstreckung zu bringen, gemeinschaftlich mit denen Warden und Inspectoren, einer jeden Ward, zwey von denen also ernannten Personen, sollen eine Woche dienen, und also nach der Reihe, in folgender Ordnung:

Für Nord-Ost Ward, Matthias Jung, John Light, Samuel Boyd, Christian Apple, Samuel Humes, John Hambrecht, Christian Petri, Jacob Mayer.

Nord-West Ward, Gottlieb Nauman, Wilhelm Reichenbach, Michael App, Abraham Deoff, Peter Bayer, Jacob Schäffer, Andreas Keiß und Ludwig Heck.

Süd-Ost Ward, Jeremias Moscher, Adam Mezzenkop, John Leitner, Leonhard Eichholz, Emanuel Reigart, John Franciscus, Henrich Pinkerten und Stoffel Franciscus.

Süd-West Ward, John Reitzel, Thomas Turner, Adam Wilhelm, Christoph Brunner, Jacob Bailey und Jacob Schwarz.

Und im Fall einige der ernannten Personen sich weigern solten zu dienen, so wird die Corporation ersucht andere an ihre Stelle zu ernennen.

Beschlossen, Daß der Corporation empfohlen werde Adam Hart und Daniel Ehler anzunehmen, welche sich an der Brücke des Herrn Abraham Witmers aufhalten sollen, um zu verhindern daß diese Schlüsse nicht gebrochen werden, und daß die Unkosten die dadurch verursacht werden, durch eine öffentliche Subscription gehoben werden sollen.

Beschlossen, Daß vorstehende Schlüsse durch Anschlagszettel publiciret werden sollen.

Jasper Yeates, Vorsizer.

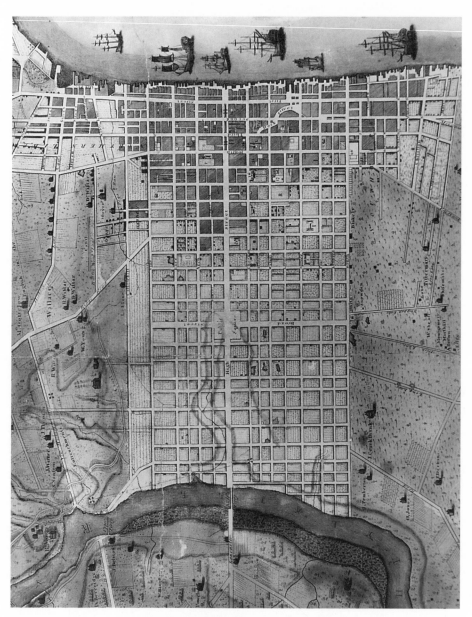

Peter C. Varlé, Plan of the City and Its Environs, 1796 (detail).
Courtesy of the Library Company of Philadelphia.

A *Melancholy Scene* of *Devastation*

The Public Response to the
1793 Philadelphia Yellow Fever Epidemic

EDITED BY

J. Worth Estes
and
Billy G. Smith

Published for the
COLLEGE OF PHYSICIANS OF PHILADELPHIA
and the
LIBRARY COMPANY OF PHILADELPHIA
by
Science History Publications/USA
1997

To the memory of Constance Coiner
"Solidarity forever"
BGS

First published in the United States of America
Science History Publications / USA
a division of Watson Publishing International
Post Office Box 493, Canton, MA 02021

Library of Congress Cataloging-in-Publication Data

A melancholy scene of devastation : the public response to the 1793 Philadelphia
  yellow fever epidemic / edited by J. Worth Estes and Billy G. Smith.
      p.   cm.
  Includes bibliographical references and index.
  ISBN 0-88135-192-X
  1. Yellow fever—Pennsylvania—Philadelphia—History—18th
century.   2. Afro-Americans—Diseases—Pennsylvania—Philadelphia—
History—18th century.   I. Estes, J. Worth, 1934–.   II. Smith, Billy G.
RC211.P5M44   1997
614.5'41'097481109033—dc21   96-54741
                                                                    CIP

Published with the assistance of the Library Company's Andrew W.
Mellon Foundation Publication Fund and a grant from the Groff Family
Memorial Trust to the College of Physicians of Philadelphia

The paper used in this publication meets the minimum requirements of the
American National Standard for Information Sciences—Permanence of Paper for
Printed Library Materials, ANSI 239.48-1984. Designed and typeset by Publishers'
Design and Production Services, Inc. Manufactured in the USA.

Contents

Contents

Foreword

N modern America, where the triumph over disease is often taken for granted and yellow fever has ceased to be a menace, it is difficult to appreciate the fear once engendered by this disease. The 1793 Philadelphia yellow fever epidemic was no mere round of sickness but a major public health emergency that paralyzed city functions, halted business and trade, and caused a breakdown in social institutions. The fever's devastating effect on what was then our nation's capital is apparent in the grim statistics it left in its wake: more than 17,000 people fled the city for safer environs, nearly 5,000 died, and hundreds of children were orphaned.

The tragic events of the 1793 Philadelphia yellow fever epidemic have been recounted in numerous works, from Mathew Carey's "instant history" to John Harvey Powell's *Bring Out Your Dead*.[1] The latter, with its dramatic portrayal of a terror-stricken city, an ill-prepared and quarrelsome medical profession, and numerous unsung heroes, remains the most useful introduction to the epidemic. Yet, despite Powell's artful prose and compelling narrative, his work has long shown its age. The essays in this volume, reflecting recent trends in social and cultural history and the history of medicine, enrich our understanding of the epidemic by investigating in greater detail the city's response and the public's reaction to the epidemic. How Philadelphia's various communities responded to the 1793 epidemic is instructive for today's urban societies, increasingly forced to deal with contagions new (AIDS) and old (tuberculosis, venereal disease).

Philadelphia's medical community was sharply divided over the fever's origin and treatment. J. Worth Estes, in his introductory essay, explains these divisions within the broader context of the complex and confused etiological and therapeutic concepts of the time. In view of the fact that a cure for yellow fever is as elusive today as it was in 1793, Estes points out that only "bed rest and supportive nursing care, along with symptomatic treatment of fever, pain, and vomiting, and perhaps correction of electrolyte imbalances" can alleviate the malady. Moreover, according to Estes, under most circumstances "only a relatively small fraction of those infected with the disease die as a result." Those who recover from yellow fever "do so largely because of what eighteenth-century physicians called the *vis medicatrix naturae*, the healing power of nature." In 1793, Estes concludes, it is probable that a large proportion of Philadelphia's citizens—anywhere from 50 to 90 percent—were infected but survived as a result of "the supporting nursing care they received as well as . . . the body's remarkable ability to heal itself, although a few may have been immune since being infected during the 1762 epidemic." What physicians could not have known in 1793 was that "none of the treatments prescribed for yellow fever could have contributed to the recovery" of any Philadelphian, "regardless of how rational, conventional, or innovative they were."

Many Philadelphians, including several physicians, used various forms of print to express their views on the yellow fever epidemic. Reflecting the recent emergence of scholarly interest in the history of printing, publishing, and reading, David Paul Nord and Sally F. Griffith present two examples of how one can achieve a better understanding of the community response to the epidemic by examining what people wrote about it.

The newspaper, according to Nord, played a crucial role during the 1793 epidemic. The *Federal Gazette*, the focus of Nord's study, became an extraordinarily important medium of information about the fever; in fact it was the only city newspaper that continued to publish throughout the epidemic. Much of the information conveyed by this newspaper, contends Nord, came not from city officials and elite physicians, but from "ordinary people, passing along rumors, offering folk cures and remedies, speculating on the religious meaning of the disease" and "sharing their fears and their sorrows." Nord's examination of the communications submitted to the *Federal Gazette* not only provides us with a better understanding of how some Philadelphians (most likely those from the "middling" and upper ranks) responded to the tragic events of 1793, but also offers us a glimpse of how an "active community of readers" sought to reconnect community bonds that were severed by the epidemic.

The concept of community is central to Sally Griffith's examination of Mathew Carey's *Short Account of the Malignant Fever*. Carey's narrative on the decline, death, and rebirth of the Philadelphia community, his first of many publishing successes, mixes a traditional admonitory interpretation of the tragic events of 1793 with an uplifting story of community regeneration resulting from the collective efforts of a virtuous citizenry. Griffith argues that Carey's account "fashioned a powerful model that helped shape the ways in which Americans responded to civic disasters, from Johnstown and Galveston in the past, to the Mississippi and Missouri valleys in the summer of 1993." Moreover, Carey's story of community rebirth through public-spirited contributions of ordinary citizens "represents a foundation narrative in civic mythology that has, in the intervening two centuries, profoundly influenced the ways that Americans have thought about their relationship to civic life in non-emergency situations."

Many of Philadelphia's physicians risked their lives during the 1793 epidemic by remaining in the city to assist the sick and dying, to serve on voluntary committees, and to work in temporary hospitals. Several died while serving their fellow citizens. Of those physicians who fought in the trenches against the dreaded malady, Benjamin Rush has become inextricably linked to the epidemic. This is due largely to the controversy that surrounded his treatment of the fever, which consisted of an aggressive regimen of bleeding and purging. Jacquelyn Miller's essay expands our understanding of Rush's controversial treatment of the disease by investigating the "multiple meanings" in his regimen. Rush, according to Miller, "assumed that the organization of social and political systems and the health of the people who populated those systems" were interconnected. Thus, Miller contends, his response to the epidemic "is best understood within the context of his larger social and politcal concerns" and should be "envisioned as a struggle to avert a second American Revolution."

The yellow fever's appearance in Philadelphia was first detected in late July. As the fever reached epidemic proportions, the city's economic life came to a halt and its social fabric disintegrated. As city authorities and the medical community struggled in their attempts to confront the crisis, Benjamin Rush appealed to Philadelphia's free blacks to assist them in the relief effort. Rush, like many of his fellow doctors, believed erroneously that blacks were immune to yellow fever and advised them that it was their duty to answer his call for help.[2] Phillip Lapsansky recounts the valiant efforts of Philadelphia's African-American community in mobilizing "the foot soldiers in the war against the epidemic." The story that Lapsansky relates is one of courage and heroism. Yet it is also a story of ingratitude and injustice on the part of Philadelphia's white community. Not only was the role of the African-American community later minimized in published accounts of the epidemic, but their noble efforts were overshadowed by charges of profiteering in Mathew Carey's best-selling account of the epidemic. In response, Absalom Jones and Richard Allen produced in 1794 *A Narrative of the Proceedings of the Black People, During the Late Awful Calamity in Philadelphia in the Year 1793 and Refutation of Some Censures, Thrown Upon Them in Some Late Publications.* The response was, in the words of Lapsansky, "the first African-American polemic, in which black leaders sought to articulate black community anger and directly confront an accuser."[3]

Much work has been done over the last two decades by historians of medicine on the history of yellow fever.[4] Recent studies by John Ellis and Margaret Humphreys on yellow fever in the American South, for example, examine how the disease influenced that region's public health movement during the nineteenth century.[5] Little work has been done, however, on Philadelphia's yellow fever epidemics and their influence on public health measures. Michal McMahon attempts to fill this gap by focusing on the struggles of city leaders and concerned citizens "to ameliorate what they believed lay behind the periodic epidemics: a filthy urban environment and a dangerously polluted water supply." This city-wide effort, argues McMahon, was the most important response to the 1793 yellow fever outbreak. He attacks the "myth" created by previous accounts of the epidemic that city government was "absent" during the crisis. While admitting that many city officials fled from the fever, McMahon contends that those who remained, together with private citizen volunteers, played an important role in addressing public health issues related to the fever. The role of city officials in shaping public health would grow in significance in the 1790s, as they joined with private citizens in mounting a community effort to devise ways to provide a clean and healthy environment for the citizens of Philadelphia.

Martin Pernick's 1972 path-breaking article on "Politics, Parties, and Pestilence," despite its age, remains the best treatment of the political response to the 1793 epidemic. Thus the editors decided to reprint it in this volume. At their request, Pernick has added a postscript in which he reexamines his arguments in light of recent scholarship, including some of the essays in this volume.

Estes's essay, which introduces the reader to the medical background of the 1793 yellow fever epidemic, is complemented nicely by Billy G. Smith's concluding comments on the papers. Whereas Estes's introduction concentrates on the etiological and therapeutic aspects of the disease, Smith's summation, which includes a concise history of yellow fever in Philadelphia, looks at the disease's social impact, particularly on the city's poor and black communities. Focusing on the theme of "community" that pervades the essays he critiques, Smith raises important questions that are pertinent to understanding the 1790s and relevant to the 1990s.

The essays we have thus far introduced succeed admirably in providing the reader with a better understanding of the city's response and the public's reaction to the 1793 epidemic. The appendices by Susan E. Klepp and Margaret Humphreys round out the volume by adding both a demographic and historiographic dimension to the story. Philadelphians who survived the crisis believed that they had lived through one of the worst afflictions ever to befall an American city, town, or community. But how bad was the 1793 epidemic, in terms of mortality? How did it compare to earlier or later epidemics? Klepp attempts to answer these questions by assessing carefully the available evidence. Klepp asserts that while the 1793 epidemic was "both terrifying and a terrible loss of human life," it "was not the worst single epidemic in

Philadelphia's history—either proportionately or absolutely." Yet, according to Klepp, though it was one of many deadly epidemics that struck the continental United States from the seventeenth through the early twentieth centuries, "this particular epidemic stands out in the collective memories of Americans." From the moment the epidemic began its retreat from their capital city, Americans searched for meaning in the tragedy. As this volume attests, the search persists.

How the 1793 Philadelphia epidemic fits into the history and historiography of yellow fever is explained by Margaret Humphreys in the volume's concluding essay. As she rightly observes, yellow fever "has become something of a growth industry in historical circles in recent years." Humphreys, a leading historian of the disease, tells us what happened to yellow fever in the United States after 1793, how and when ideas about its etiology and prevention changed, and how the essays in this volume fit into the broader historiography of the disease. Just as important, she suggests aspects of the disease that warrant further research.

The essays in this volume, with the exception of those by Martin S. Pernick, Susan E. Klepp, and Margaret Humphreys, were presented at a conference held at the College of Physicians of Philadelphia on 1 October 1993 to mark the two-hundredth anniversary of the epidemic. The conference, entitled " 'A Melancholy Scene of Devastation': The Public Response to the 1793 Philadelphia Yellow Fever Epidemic," was sponsored jointly by the College's Francis Clark Wood Institute for the History of Medicine and the Library Company of Philadelphia, and was supported with the help of grants from the Groff Family Memorial Trust and Merck & Co., Inc. The conference was organized by Thomas A. Horrocks, Director of the Francis Clark Wood Institute; James N. Green, Curator of Printed Books at the Library Company; and Gretchen Worden, Associate Director of the Francis Clark Wood Institute and Director of the Mütter Museum of the College of Physicians. Thomas Horrocks, Monique Bourque, Assistant Director for Programs in the Francis Clark Wood Institute, and John C. Van Horne, Librarian of the Library Company, were responsible for seeing this volume through press. The Groff Family Memorial Trust and the Library Company's Andrew W. Mellon Foundation Publication Fund provided subventions for this publication, which is the first in the Francis Clark Wood Institute's *Studies in the History of Medicine* series.

We wish to thank the contributors to this volume for their participation in the conference and for their cooperation and patience throughout the publication process. We owe special thanks to J. Worth Estes and Billy G. Smith for agreeing to serve as co-editors of this volume, and to those individuals who contributed to the success of the conference and to the publication of this volume: Robert H. Bradley, Jr., John M. O'Donnell, Lisa Berndt, Gretchen

Worden, Carla C. Jacobs, and Monique Bourque of the College of Physicians of Philadelphia, and James Green of the Library Company of Philadelphia. We are especially grateful to Russell C. Maulitz, Margaret Humphreys, and Susan E. Klepp for their thoughtful criticisms and helpful suggestions during the early stages of publication.

Finally, we want to express our deep appreciation to the Library Company's Andrew W. Mellon Foundation Publication Fund, the Groff Family Memorial Trust, and Merck & Co., Inc. for the grants that made the conference and the publication of this volume possible.

Philadelphia, Pennsylvania   Thomas A. Horrocks
October 1996   John C. Van Horne

NOTES

1. Mathew Carey, *A Short Account of the Malignant Fever, Lately Prevalent in Philadelphia* (Philadelphia: Mathew Carey, 1793); John H. Powell, *Bring Out Your Dead: The Great Plague of Yellow Fever in Philadelphia in 1793* (Philadelphia: University of Pennsylvania Press, 1949).
2. For information on yellow fever and mortality rates among blacks, see Kenneth Kiple and Virginia Kiple, "Black Yellow Fever Immunities, Innate and Acquired, as Revealed in the American South," *Social Science History* 1 (1977): 419–36; and Susan E. Klepp, "Seasoning and Society: Racial Differences in Mortality in Eighteenth-Century Philadelphia," *William and Mary Quarterly*, 3rd ser., 51 (1994): 473–506.
3. Jones' and Allen's *Narrative* was reprinted by Independence National Historical Park (Philadelphia) in 1993 to commemorate the two-hundredth anniversary of the 1793 Philadelphia yellow fever epidemic. See also Gary B. Nash, *Forging Freedom: The Formation of Philadelphia's Black Community, 1720–1840* (Cambridge, Mass.: Harvard University Press, 1988).
4. See Margaret Humphreys' "Yellow Fever Since 1793: History and Historiography" in this volume.
5. John H. Ellis, *Yellow Fever and Public Health in the New South* (Lexington, Ky.: The University Press of Kentucky, 1992); and Margaret Humphreys, *Yellow Fever and the South* (New Brunswick: Rutgers University Press, 1992).

Introduction: The Yellow Fever Syndrome and Its Treatment in Philadelphia, 1793

J. WORTH ESTES

HE signs and symptoms of acute infectious diseases often facilitate their recognition by both doctors and the public during epidemics. In the eighteenth century, febrile illnesses were defined by the presence of increased body heat in the first instance, although that heat was most often identified not with the aid of a thermometer but by an increased pulse rate. Fevers were then subdivided, by most observers save those who were most devoted to theoretical considerations, by the presence of regularly-spaced exacerbations. Thus, the predictable periodicity of malaria symptoms caused them to comprise the "intermittent fevers," while virtually all other febrile illnesses, in which symptoms peaked over some period of time until they reached a "crisis" and then began to wane, were usually lumped together as "continued fevers." These were further subdivided according to distinctive cutaneous features, such as jaundice, large or small pocks, petechiae (skin hemorrhages), or, if there were no such distinguishing features on the surface of the body, by the severity of the totality of their symptoms, using ill-defined adjectives such as nervous, inflammatory, or slow. Each recognizable febrile symptom was, in a sense, a different manifestation of what might be called one generic fever; no one had any idea that different species of micro-organisms cause the distinctive syndromes (and temperature fluctuation patterns) associated with the full range of febrile illnesses.[1]

The illness that struck Philadelphia from early August to late October 1793 was readily identifiable chiefly by pain in the head and abdomen, by the rapidity of its progression to death, but especially by its colors: yellow eyes and skin, purple hemorrhages into the skin, red blood pouring from the nose and mouth, and black vomit (blood that had hemorrhaged into the stomach where it had been denatured by gastric acid before being regurgitated). Many of the city's inhabitants undoubtedly came to have first-hand knowledge of the terrifying syndrome. But just to make sure, after it was all over printer

1

Mathew Carey included Dr. William Currie's clinical description of the disease in his narrative of its impact on his city. Currie's account is given here in full because the picture it presents to the mind's eye underscores and helps explain the panicky responses of both the medical profession and the public to its ravages:

> The symptoms which characterised the first stage of the fever, were, in the greatest number of cases, after a chilly fit of some duration, a quick, tense pulse—hot skin—pain in the head, back, and limbs—flushed countenance—inflamed eye—moist tongue—oppression and sense of soreness at the stomach, especially upon pressure—frequent sick qualms, and retchings to vomit, without discharging any thing, except the contents last taken into the stomach—costiveness [constipation], &c. And when stools were procured, the first generally showed a defect of bile, or an obstruction to its entrance into the intestines. But brisk purges generally altered this appearance [i.e., the stools became darker].
>
> These symptoms generally continued with more or less violence from one to three, four, or even five days; and then gradually abating, left the patient free from every complaint, except general debility. On the febrile symptoms suddenly subsiding, they were immediately succeeded by a yellow tinge in the opaque cornea, or whites of the eyes—an increased oppression at the præcordia—a constant puking of every thing taken into the stomach, with much straining, accompanied with a hoarse hollow noise.
>
> If these symptoms were not soon relieved, a vomiting of matter, resembling coffee grounds in colour and consistence, commonly called the black vomit, sometimes accompanied with, or succeeded by hæmorrhages from the nose, fauces [tonsils], gums, and other parts of the body—a yellowish purple colour, and putrescent appearance of the whole body, hiccup, agitations, deep and distressed sighing, comatose delirium, and finally death. When the disease proved fatal, it was generally between the fifth and eighth days.
>
> . . . There were, however, very considerable variations in the symptoms, as well as in the duration of its different stages. . . .
>
> In some cases, signs of putrescency appeared at the beginning, or before the end of the third day. In these, the black vomiting, which was generally a mortal symptom, and universal yellowness, appeared early. In these cases, also, a low delirium, and great prostration of strength, were constant symptoms, and coma came on very speedily.
>
> In some, the symptoms inclined more to the nervous than the inflammatory type. In these, the jaundice colour of the eye and skin, and the black vomiting, were more rare. But in the majority of cases, particularly after the nights became sensibly cooler, all the symptoms indicated violent irritation and inflammatory diathesis. In these cases, the skin was always dry, and the remissions very obscure.

The febrile symptoms, however, as has been already observed, either gave way on the third, fourth, or fifth days, and then the patient recovered; or they were soon after succeeded by a different, but much more dangerous train of symptoms, by debility, low pulse, cold skin, (which assumed a tawny colour, mixed with purple)[,] black vomiting, hæmorrhages, hiccup, anxiety, restlessness, coma, &c. Many, who survived the eighth day, though apparently out of danger, died suddenly in consequence of an hæmorrhage.[2]

Currie seems to have thought it highly important to provide all the clinical details he did, if only to emphasize their wide range of variability—or so that there would be no mistaking the accuracy of his own observations.

However, it was not only unsettling symptoms such as black vomiting, or even the possibility of death, that frightened Philadelphians in those three terrible months. So did the simple fact that the number of deaths just kept on growing. Eighteenth-century cities and towns were familiar with the usual pattern of the spread of contagious diseases among their populations that is illustrated in Figure 1, which shows the numbers of burials each day during the epidemic. Indeed, some illnesses that are not infectious were considered to be transmissible if the numbers of affected patients, or of deaths, increased steadily over time. In this case, deaths attributed to yellow fever were relatively few from 1 August until the 22nd. The steep rise from then until late October would have precluded any guesses as to when their collective affliction might end. When Mathew Carey looked at these data, in the tabular form in which he presented them in his book, he concluded that the yellow fever's "virulence may be said to have expired on the 23d, 24th, 25th, and 26th of October," and that the deaths that occurred afterward were mostly "of those long sick." Perhaps if he had graphed the data, he might have seen that the numbers of burials had actually been declining for about ten days before the 23rd.[3]

Absalom Jones and Richard Allen, two black men who had organized other blacks to nurse and bury victims of the disease, described the devastating syndrome as they had seen it. Their observations are more succinct than Currie's, but they give greater emphasis to the accompanying neurological and psychological signs. Indeed, because the nurses remained at their patients' bedsides for several days, until death or recovery, they probably had better opportunities for evaluating the full range of yellow fever victims' behavior and emotions than the doctors, who could spend only a short time with each patient they visited on their daily rounds through the stricken city:

> [Patients] were taken with a chill, a headach, a sick stomach, with pains in their limbs and back, this was the way the sickness in general began, but all were not affected alike, some appeared but slightly affected with some of these symptoms[. W]hat confirmed us in the opinion of a person

3

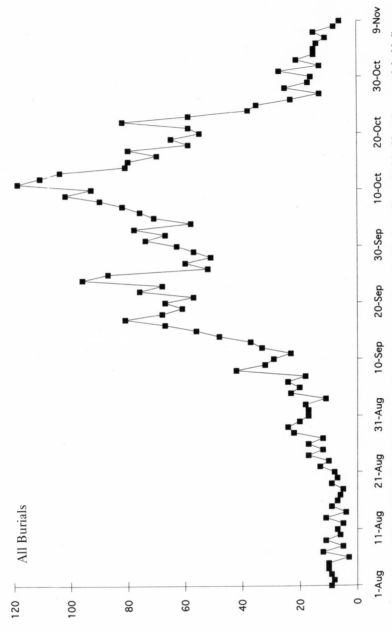

FIGURE 1. All burials in Philadelphia church graveyards, as given by Mathew Carey in his *Short Account of the Malignant Fever*, pp. 113–116. Not all of these deaths may have been direct results of infection by yellow fever, as Carey probably realized, but it would have been impossible to separate out the deaths that were not caused by the epidemic disease.

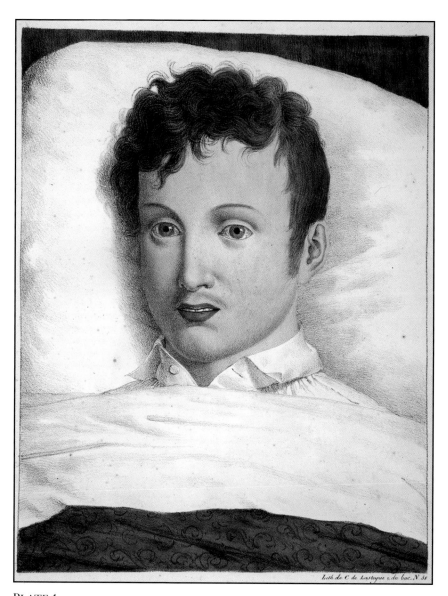

Lith de C de Lasteyrie r.du bac. N 55

PLATE 1

These are perhaps the first illustrations showing early and late stages of yellow fever in color. The first plate emphasizes the patient's red face, bloodshot eyes, and purple lips, while the second points up black vomit and nosebleed; unexpectedly, jaundice is not noticeable in either plate. Plates II and IV from [Étienne] Pariset and [André] Mazet, *Observations sur la Fièvre Jaune, Faites à Cadix, en 1819* (Paris: Audot, Libraire, 1820). Courtesy of the College of Physicians of Philadelphia.

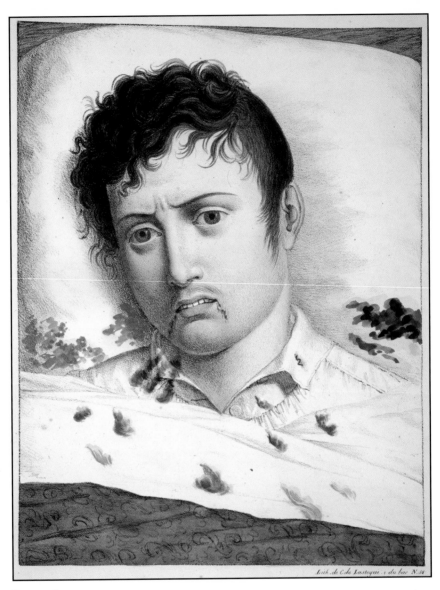

PLATE 2

being smitten was the colour of their eyes. In some it raged more furiously than in others—some have languished for seven and ten days, and appeared to get better the day, or some hours before they died, while others were cut off in one, two, or three days, but their complaints were similar. Some lost their reason and raged with all the fury madness could produce, and died in strong convulsion. Others retained their reason to the last, and seemed rather to fall asleep than die. We could not help remarking that the former were of strong passions, and the latter of a mild temper. Numbers died in a kind of dejection, they concluded they must go, (as the phrase for dying was) and therefore in a kind of fixed determined state of mind went off.[4]

Jones and Allen were not emphasizing their clinical observations, as Dr. Currie did, but they did wish to emphasize the severity of the clinical conditions they and other blacks had been called upon to nurse.

Thus, although the course of yellow fever infection varied from patient to patient, it was not difficult to diagnose once the existence of the epidemic—and its identity—had come to the attention of the medical profession and then the citizens of Philadelphia. The variable clinical course of the dramatic and highly visible illness could only have increased the public's fear of it, as is evident in some accounts of unexpected deaths (although unexpected recoveries also occurred).[5]

Indeed, some yellow fever victims may well have no symptoms at all. In others, fever up to 102°F occurs abruptly, accompanied by headache, and perhaps nausea and nosebleed, for three to four days. In many febrile illnesses, the pulse rate is proportional to body temperature. By contrast, yellow fever victims often manifest an unusual feature, a slow pulse even in the presence of a high temperature, sometimes called Faget's sign.[6] In the 1790s, physicians used the pulse in preference to a thermometer as their chief quantitative guide when assessing fevers because the pulse rate appeared to be more closely correlated with the severity of their patients' symptoms than was their thermometrically measured temperature.[7] Figure 2 illustrates Faget's sign in one of the patients that Walter Reed purposefully infected, via mosquitoes, with the yellow fever organism in 1900.

Patients who are seriously ill with yellow fever have temperatures up to 104°F or so, severe pains throughout the body, and nausea and vomiting; Faget's sign appears only after a day or two in most cases. A large proportion of victims enters remission after three days. If they do not, they then begin to develop the typical severe, classic signs of yellow fever, including jaundice, black vomit, and renal failure, during their last three to five days, followed by coma and death from liver or kidney failure, or from overwhelming infection as a result of bone marrow failure.[8] Thus, Dr. Currie's observations in 1793 are entirely consistent with modern descriptions of the disease.

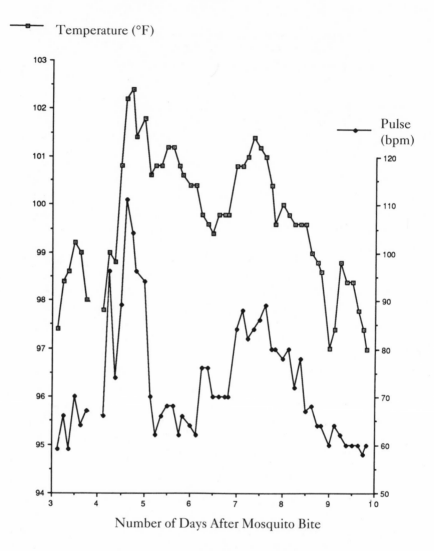

FIGURE 2. Temperature and pulse rate, measured every three hours, in case no. 6 reported by Walter Reed, Jas. Carroll, and Aristides Agramonte in "The Etiology of Yellow Fever: An Additional Note," *Journal of the American Medical Association* 36 (1901): 431–440 (reprint, 250 (1983): 649–658). Note that the pulse rose, as most eighteenth-century physicians would have expected, over the first 36 hours after the first symptoms appeared in the early morning hours of day three after the patient had been bitten by mosquitoes, and then fell (i.e., Faget's sign) to about normal rates while the thermometrically measured temperature remained over 100°F. Although the pulse did rise again, it never reached 90 beats per minute. Similar patterns are evident in the other five cases reported in the same paper.

It is important to recall that we still have no treatment that selectively counteracts or inactivates the yellow fever virus. Only bed rest and support-ive nursing care, along with symptomatic treatment of fever, pain, and vom-iting, and perhaps correction of electrolyte imbalances, can alleviate the illness. It is equally important to keep in mind that, under most circum-stances, only a relatively small fraction of those infected with the virus die as a result. Although cause-specific mortality rates as high as 20 to 70 per-cent have been recorded, the rate is most often in the range of five to ten percent. Indeed, it is difficult to be certain of the true mortality rate from yellow fever at any time, because a large fraction of those infected when they are injected with the virus by *Aedes aegypti* mosquitoes do not become sick. In short, it is nearly impossible to differentiate those who are not in-fected from those with subclinical infections.[9]

In addition, the yellow fever virus is an antigen that stimulates the forma-tion of antibodies against itself. Those who recover from the illness do so largely because of what eighteenth-century physicians called the *vis medicatrix naturae*, the healing power of nature; they were, of course, unaware of the role of the immune response. Two centuries later, it is not possible to determine the true morbidity or mortality rates of yellow fever in Philadelphia in 1793. Somewhere between eight and ten percent of the population probably suc-cumbed to it, but if the nearly half the population who fled the city are taken into account, the mortality could have been as much as 20 percent of the citi-zens at risk of infection because they remained near the mosquitoes that car-ried the virus. We can also reasonably assume that a very large proportion of citizens—anywhere from 50 to 90 percent—were infected but survived, thanks to the supportive nursing care they received as well as to the body's remarkable ability to heal itself, although a few may have been immune since being infected during an epidemic in 1762.[10]

Three factors, then—the ordinarily variable symptomatology of yellow fever, the likelihood of subclinical infections, and the antibody response to the virus—contributed to the therapeutic and social chaos in Philadelphia in the fall of 1793. By that time, most physicians and non-physicians had come to interpret the symptoms of virtually all illnesses in terms of both imbalances in the four humors and increased or decreased excitability of the body's tis-sues. By contrast, the eminent Philadelphia practitioner Dr. Benjamin Rush hypothesized—actually, he was quite certain—that all disease (not just fever) was related to excessive stimulation of the blood vessels. As a consequence, he argued, the only appropriate treatment for yellow fever victims was to re-lieve that excitement by bleeding and purging.[11] His was an oddly unique contribution to the confusion wrought by the epidemic.

Seventy years earlier, in 1724, the Reverend Cotton Mather of Boston had relied on a therapeutic logic that had been most highly developed in the Middle

Ages when he wrote that jaundice could be treated with remedies made with celandine, saffron, roasted orange, turmeric, rhubarb, gentian, and centaury—all of which have yellow pigments—along with a variety of other agents including soap, horse dung, and snails.[12] He did not specifically mention yellow fever—the term was not coined until 1750[13]—but he knew that bile, the yellow pigment of jaundice (and of urine), accumulated when the liver was diseased. In short, Mather was pointing out that the so-called "doctrine of signatures" dictated that yellow diseases could be cured with yellow drugs.

Most physicians had abandoned that notion by 1793, but they still based much of their professional thinking on the even more ancient doctrine of the four humors, which had evolved out of the Greeks' concept of the four elements. Each of the body's four humors was associated with one of the known elements: blood with fire, phlegm with water, black bile with earth, and yellow bile with air. Moreover, each humor was associated with a season of the year, and with a specific psychological effect (blood with spring and the sanguine temperament; phlegm with winter and the phlegmatic temperament; black bile with autumn and melancholy; and yellow bile with summer and the bilious or choleric temperament).

Because health was associated with the maintenance of appropriate balances among the humors, illness came to be understood as reflecting imbalances among them. As is evident in William Currie's description of yellow fever, doctors detected such imbalances at the bedside not only by the presence or absence of red, black, and yellow pigments, but also by assessing four correlate physical characteristics in the patient: heat, cold, dryness, and moisture. For 2,500 years, humoral theory had explained to everyone's satisfaction those physiological clues to the balances that had to be rectified in order to restore health and stability to the sick body. The fever that struck Philadelphia in August 1793 fit nicely into the humoral pattern, since the yellow bile that gave the febrile disease its name was associated with summer and heat. Similarly, the frequent spontaneous hemorrhages could be interpreted as the body's attempt to discharge blood that had been contaminated by foul humors, just as vomiting (whether spontaneous or drug-induced) represented the removal of noxious humors from the liver and stomach. Mather, too, had exploited humoral explanations when he wrote that emetics could remove unbalanced humors from the stomach of a jaundiced patient,[14] as was common therapeutic practice in all forms of fever. Similarly, in the 1788 edition of a popular do-it-yourself medical text that was probably known to many Philadelphians in 1793, the Reverend John Wesley recommended emetics and purges at the onset of symptoms, as well as bleeding, if the pulse is strong, to rid the body of unbalanced humors.[15]

An equally satisfying new hypothesis had gained widespread acceptance earlier in the century, largely because it was popularized by the influential fac-

ulty at Edinburgh who had trained several of Philadelphia's leading physicians. Now called the "solidist" theory, to contrast it with the older "humoral"
theory, the newer concept postulated that illness represents pathological imbalances in the irritability of the body's tissues as manifested by the tone, the
innate strength and elasticity, of the solid fibrous components of blood vessels and nerves. Both tissues were thought of as hollow tubes which propel
their respective contents through the body with forces proportional to the
tone of their constituent fibers. That is, the body was healthy when blood and
"nerve fluids" could circulate freely, or when sweat, urine, and feces could be
expelled freely, and so forth.

A fast pulse was the clinical hallmark of the generic phenomenon called
fever, because it was usually interpreted as the result of excessive stimulation
of arterial tone, requiring what was called "depletive," "sedative," or "antiphlogistic" (i.e., anti-febrile, more or less) therapy to bring it under control.
Conversely, a slow pulse was interpreted as evidence of a weakness in the fibers; it could be counteracted by stimulants, including drugs, cold water, and
electricity. Humoralism and solidism were not mutually exclusive; both concepts were used to explain the signs and symptoms of any given disease, as is
evident in Currie's description of the yellow fever syndrome, and in Jones's
and Allen's coupling of bile pigment in the eyes with the hyperactivity of the
nervous system implicit in the "madness" and convulsions they observed.

Both concepts were exploited in the design of appropriate therapy, chosen so as to fine-tune all disturbed balances simultaneously. Rush single-
handedly produced therapeutic anarchy in Philadelphia in 1793 by insisting
that yellow fever was caused solely by excessive stimulation, and by disre-
garding—or conveniently overlooking—even the possibility of diminished
stimulation at any stage of the illness.

Dr. Lionel Chalmers, of Charleston, South Carolina, had exemplified the
usual approach to fever therapy in his 1768 *Essay on Fevers*. Rush would have
agreed with Chalmers's statement that "a spasmodic contraction of the arteries is the immediate cause of fevers, and . . . the symptoms . . . are owing . . .
to an inverted or irregular circulation of the blood," even if Chalmers did focus most of his attention on fevers originating in the chest, not on yellow fever. Although his general method of treating febrile patients was like Rush's
in that it relied on purging and sweating to relieve tensions within the blood
vessels, Chalmers seldom prescribed bleeding because, he said, "much bleeding weakens the sick rather than gives lasting relief . . . and . . . the pain will
surely return, if the spasm continues."[16]

Sir John Pringle was an eminent British authority on the diseases of dense
populations, especially those of armies. He, too, associated the high temperature of yellow fever patients with arterial spasms (as assessed by measuring
the pulse rate), but he also recognized the variability in the clinical course of

the illness much as we do today. For instance, he recognized that jaundice was an unfavorable but not necessarily fatal sign, and even in epidemics, he wrote, "the mortality was not in proportion to the number of the sick, nor to the alarming nature of the symptoms." Pringle recommended that yellow fever treatment begin with bleeding, which could be repeated if its symptoms worsened, and a purge, followed by an emetic and a diaphoretic, supplemented by supportive treatment, a depletive fever regimen that resembled those used by most other physicians of the era.[17] Rush would have agreed with Pringle on the rationale for such therapy, which was designed to reduce tensions within the overstimulated febrile arterial system, although the Philadelphian administered it in exaggerated doses.

He outlined his method in the city's newspapers on 11 September so that he would not have to continue writing it out in response to endless inquiries. As soon as one felt any of the initial symptoms come on, said Rush—pain, nausea, or chills and fever—he should take ten grains of calomel and fifteen of jalap (these were far above the usual one- to two-grain doses) every six hours until the bowels had been amply evacuated several times. Rush further instructed yellow fever victims to drink fluids and lie in bed sweating. Once the bowels had been thoroughly cleansed, and if the pulse were rapid and full (as Rush thought it always was), the patient should be bled of eight or ten ounces, more if the pulse were strong enough. This basic regimen was to be accompanied by a light diet, fresh air, blisters on the sides of the body, and continued cleanliness of both body and intestines.[18]

The key to his own version of depletive therapy for yellow fever had been revealed to him in a letter that Dr. John Mitchell of Urbana, Virginia, wrote to Dr. Cadwallader Colden of New York in 1744. Benjamin Franklin sent a copy of the letter to Rush; it was published in part in 1805, and in full in 1814, after Rush's death. In it, Mitchell describes cases of yellow fever he had seen from 1737 to 1742, including several autopsies.[19]

His post-mortem observations of hemorrhage and inflammation in the gastrointestinal tract led Mitchell to conclude that the yellow fever miasma caused arterial spasms that not only resulted in inflammation of the intestines but also obstructed the flow of bile from the common bile duct into the small intestine, causing it to back up in the liver and hence into the blood, resulting in jaundice. (It should perhaps be noted here that the jaundice is now known to result from viral destruction of the liver cells that normally break down the hemoglobin in red cells into yellow bilirubin, not from blockage of the bile duct.) Mitchell postulated that the polluting miasma itself "thinned" the humors in the blood, resulting in compensatory acceleration of the pulse. Finally, he concluded that when the disturbed humors in the blood had been sufficiently heated by the fever, they caused spasms and convulsions of the arteries, exemplifying the simultaneous use of both humoral and solidist reasoning.

Mitchell went on to list six "pathognomonic symptoms" of yellow fever:

1. Sudden debility;
2. Feverish anxiety;
3. Rapid respirations (the respiratory rate was considered to be just as good as the pulse for assessing body temperature);
4. A fast pulse, followed by a slow pulse (i.e., Faget's sign) when the symptoms worsen;
5. Pain in the upper abdomen, and often in the head; and, finally,
6. Jaundice, in the eyes and skin, and even in the blood, as detected by dipping a white cloth into the serum after the blood removed by venesection has been allowed to clot.

He was probably describing his sickest yellow fever patients, which is not surprising, because it is still difficult to detect subclinical infections by the virus without relying on *in vitro* antigen-antibody reactions.

Finally, his observations at both bedside and autopsy table led Mitchell to conclude that appropriate treatment should begin with the removal of six to eight ounces of blood at the onset of mild symptoms such as headache, weakness, and vomiting, before the onset of fever. If bleeding failed to relieve the patient, he prescribed the strong emetic ipecac to remove the noxious miasma from the stomach; it would also cause sweating, which would further facilitate the removal of fouled humors from the blood. If neither treatment were successful and the full-blown fever syndrome set in, Mitchell recommended mild cathartics for speeding the removal of excess bile from the liver into the contents of the small intestine for eventual excretion in the stool. He prescribed cooling acids to dissolve the alkaline salts produced by the miasma that was contaminating the blood, and Peruvian bark (also called cinchona) to combat inflammation and restore the tone of the fibers and the state of the blood, both of which had been blighted by the yellow fever miasma. Finally, he recommended heat as adjunct stimulating therapy when the patient and his pulse had become seriously weakened.

The Virginian gained added authority in Rush's estimation because he furnished many details of autopsies he had performed. Not only did Mitchell rely on accepted humoral and solidist notions to explain the pathological effects of yellow fever on the body, but virtually all of his therapeutic notions were consistent with those of other writers on that and other fevers. However, Rush seems to have absorbed only those of Mitchell's observations that best fit his own theory of disease. Whether consciously or unconsciously, the Philadelphian did not mention the slow pulse that often characterizes yellow fever, perhaps because it does not occur at the very onset of symptoms and is a transient phenomenon. Because a physician trained at Edinburgh probably took the pulse of his febrile patients as a matter of routine, it seems likely that Rush came to his diagnostic conclusions and instituted therapy *before* the pulse fell on the second or third day of his patients' symptoms (see Figure 2). Besides, even if he had waited a day or two before instituting treatment, a slow pulse would have been inconsistent with his theory that all disease was secondary to excessive stimulation of the vessels, and so could be disregarded.

The linchpins of Rush's yellow fever therapy were bleeding and large doses of jalap, which causes catharsis, and calomel (mercurous chloride), which induces emesis and diuresis as well as catharsis. These clear-cut effects provided good evidence that the drugs had indeed relieved the body of the foul humors produced by the yellow fever miasma. At the same time, Rush thought his depletive remedies would relieve the intravascular tensions which he believed to be the cause of his patients' symptoms. As he saw it, his major contribution to the treatment of yellow fever stemmed from his recognition that Mitchell had not prescribed *sufficient* amounts of bleeding, calomel, or jalap.[20]

Although some of the many physicians who treated Philadelphians afflicted during the epidemic followed Rush's recommendations, others employed more conventional fever remedies. For instance, William Currie began with tartar emetic (antimony potassium tartrate), until the patient either purged or vomited. The next day he gave a milder purge, and a diaphoretic to encourage sweating. He agreed with Rush as to the extent to which it was necessary to calm overstimulated vessels, which suggests that he may not have observed Faget's sign, but he seldom bled his yellow fever patients because, he said, they were already too debilitated. He prescribed other remedies as needed, such as Peruvian bark and laudanum (tincture of opium), when he thought the patient was ready for them.[21] That is, his overall *modus curandi* was far milder than Rush's.

A French physician in Philadelphia, David Nassy, may have observed Faget's sign inasmuch as he reported that the pulse rate was not proportional to body temperature in his own yellow fever patients. This seems to have been one of the factors that led him to avoid adopting a depletive therapeutic program as rigorous as Rush's. Nassy did prescribe bleeding, emetics, and cathartics at the onset of symptoms, as did Rush, Isaac Cathrall, and other Philadelphia practitioners, but in smaller doses, tailoring his remedies to each patient's special needs. Adam Kuhn favored an even milder variant of the same method, prescribing cathartics only for patients who were constipated, although both he and Nassy took pains not only to strengthen patients who had been weakened by yellow fever but also to try to minimize the degree of their debilitation in the first place.[22]

Jean Devèze, the French physician who ran the Bush Hill hospital for indigent victims of the epidemic, had arrived from Santo Domingo (now Haiti) in July. Because he had had considerable experience with yellow fever in the

12

West Indies, he thought that its victims required gentle remedies and pleas-ant surroundings to assist the *vis medicatrix naturae*, not fight it, as strong depletive measures did. He, too, prescribed stimulants, including Peruvian bark, for weak patients, but not bleeding. Devèze and Nassy autopsied sev-eral yellow fever victims on the latter's initiative. Their post-mortem observa-tions, Nassy reported, "have plainly proved the havoc that those violent medicines [i.e., those prescribed by Rush], when administered in an inflam-matory sickness, have caused in the stomach and intestines."[23] It is difficult to know if this inference was correct, since yellow fever itself causes extensive damage to the intestinal mucosa, but to the French-trained physicians it was one more clue to the hazards of Rush's notoriously harsh treatment.

The medical community of Philadelphia was as sharply divided over the source of yellow fever as it was over what constituted effective therapy. Some, like Rush and Devèze, believed that the affected body's balances were dis-rupted by a miasma or effluvium that arose from local sources of decay and spread through the air until it disturbed the humors and tones of the bodies it entered. Others, like Currie, argued that it was a contagion that was transmit-ted from person to person. But John Redman Coxe, a pupil of Rush's in 1793, recalled many years later that "Experiments were made [he did not say by whom] by swallowing the black vomit, or by inoculating with it with perfect impunity; not a solitary instance could be adduced in favor of contagion!"[24] Mathew Carey shared the opinion of many that the epidemic had been brought from the West Indies, probably on the ships that, since early July, had brought 2,000 refugees (including Dr. Devèze) who were fleeing the outbreak of a violent slave revolt in Santo Domingo. Carey also collected data which, to his surprise, showed that the prevalence of yellow fever was not affected by the weather.[25] Although there were strong political correlates of the physi-cians' opinions on how the disease had spread through the city, that di-chotomy did not spill over into the debate over appropriate therapy.[26]

It is clear that none of the treatments prescribed for yellow fever could have contributed to the recovery of any Philadelphian in those terrible three months in 1793, regardless of how rational, conventional, or innovative they were. Most of the city's doctors based their favorite therapies on clinical ob-servations made at their patients' bedsides, rooting them within the time-tested framework of humoral and solidist thinking. It might have been thought that Rush disregarded or simply missed the peculiar behavior of the pulse rate in this fever, that he based his conclusion that his treatment was efficacious solely on his patients' recoveries, permitting him to exclaim, in prideful exultation, that he had demonstrated "the triumph of a principle in medicine."[27]

However, he was probably not completely blind to what later observers la-beled Faget's sign. That is, as a graduate of the medical school of Edinburgh, where the pulse was routinely counted on the teaching wards, he almost certainly measured it when assessing his febrile patients.[28] Thus, the reduction of the pulse rate a day or two after he had administered his standard treatment of purging and bleeding could only have confirmed his opinion of its merits as depletive or antiphlogistic therapy. However, it is not likely that his patients would have benefited any more than they did from his ministrations even if he had recognized the anomaly.

Because many people who are infected with the yellow fever virus either develop no symptoms or recover from those they do display, it is not possible to evaluate retrospectively the success or failure of the yellow fever remedies prescribed by Rush, Devèze, Currie, other members of the College of Physicians of Philadelphia, or anyone else, for that matter. That is, none left behind any surviving notes that are even remotely analogous to data from modern clinical trials. Rush did inadvertently provide a few data in the form of news about friends and civic notables that he passed on to his wife and other correspondents in the many letters he wrote during the panic. Out of 50 of his own yellow fever patients that have been identified by name in those letters, 39 (78%) recovered. Altogether, he mentioned recovery or death of 72 named fever patients, but only the 50 are known with certainty to have been under his care; all of the other 22 died.[29] In the end, no Philadelphia doctor had any reason to abandon whatever therapy he favored, sometimes after a modest trial period. Any of them may have been disappointed with the efficacy of the method he chose, but each was confident that he was doing the right thing for the right reason. As it was put by one of the three physicians who bled George Washington to death six years later, "we thought we were right, and so we are justified."[30]

The following essays relate the responses of several segments of the citizenry of Philadelphia to the onslaught of the disturbingly colorful symptoms that make up yellow fever, in the context of the political and cultural circumstances of the fledgling American republic in 1793. At the same time, they underscore the theoretical battles among the city's physicians, the uselessness of their medicines, and the uniquely beneficial role of nursing in facilitating recovery from a disease that everyone could recognize for what it was—a terrifying threat to life, liberty, and the pursuit of happiness in the new republic, in all the meanings of those words inferred by the inhabitants of the nation's first capital city, from its physicians to its artisans, intellectuals, merchants, politicians, technocrats, blacks and whites, rich and poor—a cross-section of urban America in the 1790s.

Acknowledgment: I am grateful to Reagan Quan for constructing the graphs for the two figures.

NOTES

1. J. Worth Estes, "Quantitative Observations of Fever and its Treatment Before the Advent of Short Clinical Thermometers," *Medical History* 35 (1991): 189–216. Although my outline is rather simplified, the interested reader can begin to find how theories appeared, flourished, and competed among themselves in the essays presented in W. F. Bynum and V. Nutton, eds., *Theories of Fever from Antiquity to the Enlightenment* (London: Wellcome Institute for the History of Medicine, 1981). For one careful observer's definitions of individual syndromes, see John Huxham, *An Essay on Fevers*, 3rd ed. (1757; reprint, Canton, Mass.: Science History Publications, 1988).

2. Mathew Carey, *A Short Account of the Malignant Fever, Lately Prevalent in Philadelphia*, 4th ed. (Philadelphia: Mathew Carey, 1794), pp. 13–14.

3. Ibid., p. 64. For an example of a non-contagious disease (scurvy) that was thought to be contagious, see J. Worth Estes, "A Naval Surgeon in the Barbary Wars: Dr. Peter St. Medard on New York, 1802–1803," in *New Aspects of Naval History*, eds. Department of History, U.S. Naval Academy (Baltimore: Nautical and Aviation Publishing Co. of America, 1985), pp. 81–92.

4. A[bsalom] J[ones] and R[ichard] A[llen], *A Narrative of the Proceedings of the Black People, during the Late Awful Calamity in Philadelphia, in the Year 1793: And a Refutation of Some Censures, Thrown upon Them in Some Late Publications* (1794; reprint, Philadelphia: Franklin Court Print Shop & Bindery, 1979), p. 21.

5. John H. Powell, *Bring Out Your Dead* (Philadelphia: University of Pennsylvania Press, 1949; reprint, New York: Time, Inc., 1965, and reprint, Philadelphia: University of Pennsylvania Press, 1993), passim. This book is essential reading on the epidemic.

6. Donald B. Cooper and Kenneth F. Kiple, "Yellow Fever," in *The Cambridge World History of Human Disease*, ed. Kenneth F. Kiple (New York: Cambridge University Press, 1993), pp. 1100–1107.

7. J. Worth Estes, "Drug Usage at the Infirmary: The Example of Dr. Andrew Duncan, Sr.," Appendix D to Guenter B. Risse, *Hospital Life in Enlightenment Scotland: Care and Teaching at the Royal Infirmary of Edinburgh* (New York: Cambridge University Press, 1986), pp. 351–384; Estes, "Quantitative Observations." Because many leading Philadelphia physicians, including Rush, had been trained at Edinburgh, they usually followed their preceptors' example in this respect as in others; see, for instance, Whitfield J. Bell, Jr., "Medicine in Boston and Philadelphia: Comparisons and Contrasts," in *Medicine in Colonial Massachusetts, 1620–1820*, eds. Philip Cash, Eric H. Christianson, and J. Worth Estes (Boston: Colonial Society of Massachusetts, 1980), pp. 159–183, esp. 164, 167, 171–173; and, for Rush, Robert B. Sullivan, "Sanguine Practices: A Historical and Historiographic Reconsideration of Heroic Therapy in the Age of Rush," *Bulletin of the History of Medicine* 68 (1994): 211–234.

8. Jay P. Sanford, "Arbovirus Infections," in *Harrison's Principles of Internal Medicine*, eds. Jean D. Wilson et al., 12th ed., 2 vols. (New York: McGraw-Hill, Inc., 1991), 1: 725–739; the description of yellow fever is on pp. 734–735.

9. Ibid.; Cooper and Kiple, "Yellow Fever."

10. It has been difficult to estimate the death rates in Philadelphia in late 1793 with any precision even from the data given by Mathew Carey in his *Short Account*, pp. 113–116 (see Figure 1), or from those reprinted by Susan E. Klepp in her monumental

compilation, *The Swift Progress of Population: A Documentary and Bibliographic Study of Philadelphia's Growth, 1642–1859* (Philadelphia: American Philosophical Society, 1991), pp. 51–52, 79. I am grateful to Dr. Klepp for providing me with her unpublished summary of all the available data; see also Klepp's essay in this volume. Carey counted 4,041 burials of people who died of all causes from 1 August through 9 November, about eight percent of the total population. (Thus, it is possible, even if not likely, that the entire population of Philadelphia could have been infected with yellow fever virus in 1793.) During the six years before 1793, the average number of deaths from all causes recorded annually was approximately 1,180; thus, in the normal course of events one would have expected about 325 deaths during that time span (or perhaps a few more, since late summer often heralded the onset of increased mortality from certain infections throughout the country). Powell estimated the total deaths at over 5,000 (*Bring Out Your Dead*, p. 302) and Klepp agrees; this seems reasonable inasmuch as the fates of many citizens who fled the city are unknown, and many more deaths were undoubtedly unrecorded. Regardless of the imprecision of calculated death or cause-specific death rates for the time, the few numbers available make clear the devastation that yellow fever wrought on Philadelphia in late 1793, especially in its most densely populated areas. John Duffy (*Epidemics in Colonial America* [Baton Rouge: Louisiana State University Press, 1953], p. 152) raised the possibility that the 1762 epidemic was dengue, which would not have affected the immune response to yellow fever in 1793, although all contemporary observers called the earlier disease yellow fever.

11. The fullest outline of Rush's theory is in his *Medical Inquiries and Observations*, 2nd ed., 4 vols. (Philadelphia: J. Conrad and Co., 1805), 3: 3–66. It and the supporting data he cites deserve fuller analysis, in the light of eighteenth-century concepts of physiology, than can be given here. His 1794 *Account of the Bilious Remitting Yellow Fever, as It Appeared in the City of Philadelphia, in the Year 1793*, appears on pp. 67–353 of *Medical Inquiries*; he had not changed his mind about his treatment of yellow fever victims in the intervening twelve years.

12. Cotton Mather, *The Angel of Bethesda* (MSS., 1724; first published Barre, Mass.: American Antiquarian Society and Barre Publishers, 1972), pp. 191–195.

13. Cooper and Kiple, "Yellow Fever."

14. Mather, *Angel of Bethesda*, pp. 191–195.

15. John Wesley, *Primitive Physic; Or, an Easy and Natural Method of Curing Most Diseases*, 22nd ed. (London: The New Chapel, 1788), p. 60.

16. Lionel Chalmers, *An Essay on Fevers* (London: Edward and Charles Dilly, 1768), pp. 42–54.

17. Sir John Pringle, *Observations on the Diseases of the Army*, 7th ed. (London: W. Strahan, J. and F. Rivington, W. Johnston, T. Payne, T. Longman, Wilson and Nicoll, T. Durham, and T. Cadell, 1775), pp. 169–172, 181, 210, 220–221; Estes, "Drug Usage at the Infirmary." For the sequence in which remedies were administered, see also J. Worth Estes, "Naval Medicine in the Age of Sail: The Voyage of the *New York*, 1802–1803," *Bulletin of the History of Medicine* 56 (1982): 238–253.

18. Powell, *Bring Out Your Dead*, p. 139. For a typical light, or "low," diet such as Rush might have prescribed, see J. Worth Estes, *Dictionary of Protopharmacology: Therapeutic Practices 1700–1850* (Canton, Mass.: Science History Publications, 1990), pp. 66–67.

19. John Mitchell, "Account of the Yellow Fever which Prevailed in Virginia in the Years 1737, 1741, and 1742, in a Letter to the Late Cadwallader Colden, Esq. of New-York," *American Medical & Philosophical Register* 4 (1814): 181–215. Duffy (*Epidemics*, p. 152) suggested that these Virginia epidemics, too, might have been dengue, although the evidence is less compelling here than for Philadelphia in 1762; besides, in this case it would not matter, since Rush accepted Mitchell's diagnosis of yellow fever. For Rush's enlightenment by Mitchell, see the latter's *Medical Inquiries*, pp. 227–229. For the correlation between respiratory rate and temperature—Mitchell's symptom no. 3—see also Estes, "Quantitative Observations." For definitions of the specific drugs mentioned throughout this essay, see Estes, *Dictionary*.

20. Rush, *Medical Inquiries*, pp. 231–257. It should not be assumed that Rush's therapeutic method was illogical. For instance, he reasoned that "The jalap appeared to be a necessary addition to [calomel], in order to quicken its passage through the bowels; for calomel is slow in its operation, most especially when it is given in large doses" (ibid., p. 231). Moreover, he prescribed bleeding, cold water, and several other remedies "to abstract excess of stimulus [that is, the miasma that causes the arterial system to display the symptoms of yellow fever] from the system" (ibid., p. 233).

21. William Currie, *A Description of the Malignant Fever Prevailing at Present in Philadelphia* (Philadelphia: Thomas Dobson, 1793), pp. 16–22.

22. D[avid] Nassy, *Observations on the Cause, Nature, and Treatment of the Epidemic Disorder, Prevalent in Philadelphia*, trans. from French (Philadelphia: Parker and Co., for Mathew Carey, 1793), pp. 17–19; Powell, *Bring Out Your Dead*, pp. 76–77.

23. Nassy, *Observations*, p. 24; Powell, *Bring Out Your Dead*, pp. 162–174.

24. Powell, *Bring Out Your Dead*, pp. 37–46; Jack Eckert, "In the Days of the Epidemic: The 1793 Yellow Fever Outbreak in Philadelphia as Seen by Physicians," *Transactions & Studies of the College of Physicians of Philadelphia*, Ser. 5, 15 (1993): 31–38.

25. Powell, *Bring Out Your Dead*, pp. 4–5; Carey, *Short Account*, pp. 67–70, 113–116.

26. Martin S. Pernick, "Politics, Parties, and Pestilence: Epidemic Yellow Fever in Philadelphia and the Rise of the First Party System," reprinted and updated in the present volume.

27. Rush, *Medical Inquiries*, p. 234. Rush did, however, note that the pulse could be as low as 30 to 60 beats per minute, due to the "stimulus of the remote cause acting upon the arteries with too much force to admit of their being excited into quick and convulsive motions" (ibid., p. 98), an explanation which probably fell on deaf ears at the time, but his descriptions of his own yellow fever patients suggest that those with such low pulse rates were in or near shock (perhaps hypovolemic).

28. Estes, "Drug Usage at the Infirmary." It should be noted that bleeding *per se* does not reliably diminish the pulse rate to any extent, despite what has been reported in the past; see Estes, "Quantitative Observations."

29. Chris Holmes, "Benjamin Rush and the Yellow Fever," *Bulletin of the History of Medicine* 40 (1966): 246–263.

30. J. T. Howard, "The Doctors Gustavus Brown: Father and Son, of Charles County, Maryland," *Annals of Medical History*, n.s., 9 (1937): 427–448.

Readership as Citizenship in Late-Eighteenth-Century Philadelphia

DAVID PAUL NORD

N the early morning darkness of 8 September 1793, the cry of "Fire!" rang out in Philadelphia. One man, awakened by the alarm, hesitated to leave his house to join the bucket brigades. He was momentarily frozen in fear that death lay waiting for him in the streets of the city, for in the autumn of 1793 Philadelphia was gripped by epidemic yellow fever. Quickly, however, he overcame his fear and resolved to do his duty:

> What, thought I, is to become of us at this critical moment, amid the sickness which is now prevailing? I knew, however, that exertions would be necessary, and believed it right for me to turn out and use my efforts, which notwithstanding the numerous probable obstacles at such a juncture, I had no doubt would be in conjunction with a considerable number of the remaining citizens. I prepared myself according to the best of my judgment for the occasion; I bathed my temples and forehead with the proper vinegar, took some in my mouth, and went forward....
>
> While I was occupied handing buckets, I looked at my companions on each side, but did not know them; they might for anything I knew, have come from the gloomy chambers of debilitated friends or relatives; I stayed, however, at my post as long as it appeared necessary, and then went home. After writing the chief part of what precedes, I ate my breakfast....[1]

This man's story is revealing in several ways. It suggests something about the nature of community life in an increasingly impersonal city, a place where strangers, caught up in common disasters, might meet, in bucket lines and elsewhere. It also suggests something about the importance that writing held for this man in his efforts to make sense of his experience: He wrote his narrative, then he ate his breakfast. But the most interesting aspect of the story may not be what it says about civic virtue or about this man's need to write out his thoughts. Perhaps most interesting is that, the next day, he sent his story to a newspaper.

Why would someone send an anonymous personal narrative such as this to a newspaper? Why would someone send anything to a newspaper during a catastrophe such as the yellow fever epidemic? Surely the answer is that people sent material to newspapers because they believed other people would profit from reading it or would simply enjoy reading it. A study of the correspondence sent to late-eighteenth-century newspapers, therefore, should reveal what some readers thought other readers should read. This is especially true, I believe, of newspaper correspondence submitted during a community crisis, such as the Philadelphia yellow fever epidemic. During this crisis, the newspaper (indeed, a single newspaper, the *Federal Gazette*) became an extraordinarily important medium of public communication. The paper brimmed with information about the fever. And much of this information came not from public officials, but from the people of the city—the readers of the newspaper.

This essay, then, is a study of the civic function of the newspaper during the yellow fever crisis in Philadelphia in 1793. But not only that. The correspondence in the newspaper (and commentary on newspaper reading in contemporary letters and diaries) opens a window on the readers of the newspaper as well. These correspondents were readers writing for other readers, and the material they shared with each other is a fascinating collection of evidence for the history of reading.[2] What was the public purpose of reading the newspaper in the late-eighteenth-century American city? That is the question that this essay will explore.

From the beginning, observers saw the role of the newspaper, especially the *Federal Gazette*, as crucial to the public response to the yellow fever epidemic. In his instant history of the epidemic, Mathew Carey proclaimed the *Federal Gazette* "of utmost service in conveying to the citizens of the United States authentic intelligence of the state of the disorder, and of the city." Most historians who have written about the yellow fever have followed Carey in assigning to the newspaper the rather simple role of information disseminator.[3] My approach is somewhat different. I am interested in the readers, a very active community of readers, who gathered around the *Federal Gazette* during the fearful autumn of 1793.[4] This reader community included city officials and elite physicians who sought to commandeer the paper to disseminate their own versions of "authentic intelligence." But it also included ordinary people passing along rumors, offering folk cures and remedies, speculating on the religious meaning of the disease, and sharing their fears and their sorrows. For all of these people, the newspaper was a place for community participation, and readership a form of citizenship.[5]

THE SETTING

> [Through newspapers] we keep company with the absent; we are, by
> their means made acquainted with strangers—we feel, in solitude, a sym-
> pathy with mankind.[6]

When the man in the fire bucket line looked to his left and right, he saw
strangers. That scene symbolizes Philadelphia's changing community life in
1793. No longer was Philadelphia "a single community," as Sam Bass Warner
has characterized it in its pre-Revolutionary days.[7] By 1793, Philadelphia had
become the metropolis of North America, a complex urban center controlling
nearly one-quarter of the export trade of the United States, housing both state
and federal governments, and teeming with a population of some 51,000.[8]
The gap between the rich and poor, always wide, was probably growing wider
in the 1790s, as rents escalated, as immigration increased, and as an economic
system based upon the harsh insecurities of wage labor took root. More than
half of the families owned no real property at all, and one-third probably lived
at the subsistence level.[9] This class division was increasingly manifest as residential division as well. By 1793, the compact, mixed-class eighteenth-century town was disappearing, as the poor settled on the periphery, reserving
the older core wards for the rich. Taken together, these economic and social
transformations prompted one contemporary observer to call Philadelphia
"one great hotel or place of shelter for strangers."[10]

Yet Philadelphia remained a community. Men still turned out to fight a
neighbor's fire and, if necessary, an epidemic. Gary Nash has urged historians
of eighteenth-century cities to pay closer attention to the new forms of community life that took root in the rubble of the old. "Rather than nostalgically
tracing the eclipse of community," he says, "we need to trace the continu-
ously evolving process of community." He talks of the growth of working-
class taverns and craft organizations, middle- and upper-class benevolent and
reform associations, and (his special interest) free black churches and self-help
societies. Far from dismissing these formal, structured organizations as mere
gesellschaft, Nash assigns to them a leading role in the creation of true urban
community, of what he calls "'gemeinschaft of mind'—the mental life of the
community."[11]

In other words, the increasing complexity of the modern city required formal structures to build community and to hold it together. For Nash, the most
interesting of these formal structures are working-class political movements
and voluntary associations—structures that helped groups of urban people
fabricate their own "communities within communities."[12] For me, the most
interesting of these structures are those that sought to maintain a city-wide

sense of community. And these structures have frequently been the institutions of public communication and—for literate people—of print.[13]

As community life in the city became more complex and more formally structured, so did the communication system. In his discussion of the community life of pre-revolutionary Philadelphia, Sam Bass Warner links community to communication; but in his account communication was almost entirely oral and interpersonal, swirling through the streets, taverns, and families of the city. Though Philadelphia had two newspapers and a prosperous publishing trade by the early 1760s, Warner does not think it necessary to mention printing in his discussion of the city's "communications system."[14] Such an omission would be strikingly inappropriate for the 1790s. The revolution and its aftermath left Philadelphians with a heightened taste for newspaper reading. By 1794, the city had eight newspapers, four of them dailies. (The first dailies in America appeared in Philadelphia in the 1780s.) These newspapers carried at least ten times as much material as had the city's two weeklies in 1764. Meanwhile, the proportion of space given over to local news, compared with foreign and national news, was growing as well—from 12 percent to 23 percent of the total news space. The circulation of most of these newspapers is unknown, though likely none was more than 1,500. So, newspaper reading was certainly not a universal experience for all classes of Philadelphians in the 1790s. Indeed, some small but considerable proportion of Philadelphians could not read in 1793, though the exact illiteracy rate is also unknown.[15] But newspaper reading was common enough to lead one smug and successful Philadelphia publisher to declare, in verse, that the newspaper was "everyone's hobby horse":

We say (with deference to the college)
News Papers are the spring of knowledge;
The gen'ral source throughout the nation,
Of every modern conversation.[16]

One such "spring of knowledge" in 1793 was Andrew Brown's *Federal Gazette and Philadelphia Daily Advertiser*, a successful and fairly typical Philadelphia daily. Brown had been the principal of a girls' academy before he launched the *Federal Gazette* in 1788 to plump for the new constitution; and like many of his fellow republican educators, he held to the belief that in popular knowledge lay the stability of government and the safety of the people. "The foundation of all free governments seems to be a general diffusion of knowledge," he wrote. Like his fellow editors, Brown came to associate the success of newspapers with the progress of republican government and the success of the American experiment. In the self-congratulatory rhetoric that newspaper publishers loved then and still love today, Brown ranked newspapers with schools as "heralds of truth" and "protectors of peace and good order"; and he proclaimed his own paper "a faithful guardian of the sacred rights of the community."[17]

For Andrew Brown, the function of the newspaper at the local level was a blend of community booster and community forum. In his first issue, he published a list of projects that a proper newspaper should pursue, including "the advancement of agriculture, manufactures, and commerce in and around Philadelphia." This booster spirit remained part of the *Federal Gazette*'s publicly stated mission.[18] At the same time, Brown promised that his paper would be open to all correspondents. Though committed to the federal constitution and the Republican interpretation of it, the *Federal Gazette* was not intended by Brown to be a party paper. He insisted that by "free press" he meant a newspaper "open to writers on both sides of every political or other question."[19] Like several of the other large dailies in Philadelphia in the 1790s (such as John Dunlap's *American Daily Advertiser*), Brown's *Federal Gazette* seemed to make its way more as a community common carrier than as a party organ. In a paean to community-building, Brown declared of newspapers:

> We keep company with the absent; we are, by their means, made acquainted with strangers—we feel, in solitude, a sympathy with mankind. . . . Men stick to their business, and yet the public is addressed as a town meeting. Yet the gazettes follow us to our closets and give us counsel there.[20]

This is not to suggest that Brown conducted the *Federal Gazette* as a kind of public philanthropy. Not at all. The *Federal Gazette* was a decidedly private business. Even in his public statements, Brown made this clear. He seldom failed to remind his readers that his good service to the community warranted their financial support, through subscriptions and advertising.[21] Moreover, there is some evidence from inside the business to suggest that Brown may have been a quintessential private enterpriser. One of his apprentices, Robert Simpson, described him as "a very wicked man" and "a vile monster," who beat his apprentices, fed them scraps, and forced them to work on the Sabbath in order to squeeze from the business as much personal gain as possible. "However he may flourish in this life," Simpson wrote to a runaway apprentice friend, "he will one day or other receive the punishment so justly his due."[22]

The *Federal Gazette*, then, was a private institution, but one clothed in public purpose. In 1793, when the yellow fever began to spread, people turned to the newspaper, this newspaper. They turned to it to get information; they also turned to it to give information. The resentful Robert Simpson may have been correct to assume that Andrew Brown's motives for staying in business during the fever were purely pecuniary. But, regardless of Brown's private motives, Philadelphians seemed to agree that the *Federal Gazette* played a key public role in the community's response to the epidemic.[23] Indeed, many probably agreed entirely with Brown's own boast "that the continued publication of this paper amid scenes of uncommon danger and daily threatening mortality, has been of great use to the public. It has kept whole the general chain of intelligence that must otherwise have been broken."[24] But what was this "chain of intelligence"? What kind of community institution or forum should a newspaper be? What sort of civic function should newspaper publishing and newspaper reading serve? On these questions, agreement was less than complete.

THE FEVER

Their burying grounds are like ploughed fields.[25]

The story began quietly in the late summer of 1793. A few cases of an unusually malignant fever appeared near Water Street. The symptoms were severe: fever and chills, a feeble pulse, deep torpor, delirium, a morbid yellowing of the skin and eyes, a fetid black vomit. As their patients died, one by one, the physicians of Philadelphia worried and conferred. The most famous among them, Dr. Benjamin Rush, recalled the visitation of a similar fever in Philadelphia in 1762. On 19 August, he was prepared to call this new pestilence by name: the yellow fever. As the death toll mounted, the doctors despaired, for, as Rush wrote to his wife in late August, the disease mocked the best efforts of medicine.[26]

By the end of August, panic was building in Philadelphia. Thousands fled. Those who stayed shuttered themselves into their houses. The few who ventured out buried their mouths and noses in vinegar-soaked handkerchiefs. By September the streets of the city were largely abandoned to the carters of the dead and dying. The ordeal lasted through October, and in its course more than 4,000 died.[27] The epidemic seemed to crush the survivors as well. In his account of the fever, Mathew Carey described case after case of tragedy and terror. He concluded that "while affairs were in this deplorable state, and people at the lowest ebb of despair, we cannot be astonished at the frightful scenes that were acted, which seemed to indicate a total dissolution of the bonds of society."[28]

Of course, the bonds of society were not dissolved. As Carey himself acknowledged, the fever produced scenes of bravery as well as panic, heroism as well as cruelty, community organization as well as chaos.[29] It also produced an incredible rush of communication—the fundamental bond of society. The fever dominated every channel of communication within Philadelphia and between Philadelphia and the outside world, from word-of-mouth rumor to learned medical treatise. But one channel—the newspaper—seems to have taken on a particularly important community role. Nearly everyone, from public officials to letter writers and diarists, seems to have turned to it. Even the doggerel poet of the fever, Samuel Stearns, acknowledged his debt to the newspaper:

A pestilence, which there did rage
With rapid force, has swept away
An hundred people from the stage,
Within the compass of a day.
But sometimes less, and sometimes more,
The daily publications tell,
Upon that mournful city's shore,
In that short time, have often fell.[30]

Though the newspaper was in some ways "the source of every modern conversation" during the fever, people had very different ideas of what it should do. Some believed that it should be the voice of authority, a font of what Mathew Carey called "authentic intelligence." Others believed that it should be the conversation of community, a forum for "every observation" on the fever.

"AUTHENTIC INTELLIGENCE"

The hundred tongues of rumor were never more successfully employed than on this melancholy occasion.[31]

The yellow fever dominated the private conversations of Philadelphians and of those with links to Philadelphia. The surviving letters and diaries overflow with the news.[32] Of course, much of the news was nothing more than rumor, and many of these rumors were printed in newspapers all over the country. This flood of rumors, both private and public, exasperated the authorities of Philadelphia. The public officials and the leading physicians believed that the spread of rumor—especially in the newspapers—contributed mightily to the distress of the city.[33] Letter writers were exasperated as well. Their correspondence is filled with warnings to friends and loved ones not to believe the wild rumors they might hear.[34] But as an antidote to rumor, both private citizens and public authorities turned to the same medium that seemed most recklessly effective in spreading rumor: the newspaper.

The letters and diaries suggest that news spread mainly by word of mouth and letter. "This day's mail brings us dismal accounts indeed from your metropolis," one New Yorker wrote to relatives in Philadelphia. He urged his

25

brother-in-law to write to the family in New York by at least every other post, because "so many dreadful and contradictory reports prevail here that we know not what to believe."[35] As far away as London, stories of the epidemic were circulated by travelers and letters, and anxious relatives waited and worried. Closer to Philadelphia, the distress was all consuming. "My thoughts are full of the subject," a young woman wrote to her father. "It is difficult to disengage them to obtain even that momentary relief that seems necessary to health."[36] But the news was inescapable: "Anxiously did I wait the time for the post to arrive each day, but alas everyday brought more distressing accounts and made me even dread to hear."[37] And as the news was dreadful but inescapable, so was the need to spread it. In a long, clumsy letter to his brother, a young Philadelphia artisan spilled out the story, adding "I had no expectations when I begun this letter, to have made it so lengthy, but being led on from one thought, to another, it seems almost impossible to stop."[38]

The scene in nearby Germantown provides a glimpse of how the news system worked. Thousands of Philadelphians fled to the outlying towns, especially Germantown, to weather the storm. There they waited, hungry for news. Elizabeth Drinker's diary is filled with reports from the city, usually brought out by traveler or letter. Her entries for these doleful days are replete with the vague attributions of second-hand news: "we have heard this day," "we have an account this morning," "several carriages stopped to talk," "they say they have received a letter or letters," "some say," "it is said." The entries are also filled with skepticism. "The accounts this day from the city are many and various," she writes, but they "are not ascertained." She tells of "hearsays from the city of a great number of funerals," but she hopes that "the number is greatly exaggerated." She mentions rumors that Negroes may have poisoned the wells, but "those are flying reports, and most likely false."[39] Another diarist, Jacob Hiltzheimer, who stayed in Philadelphia, describes the nervous ambivalence of the refugees: "Rode out to Germantown, which is filled with Philadelphians who were anxious to hear the news from the city, but kept their distance when they found we were from there."[40]

Although people depended heavily on private communication for information about the fever, many turned to the newspapers for a kind of authentication of the news. Susanna Dillwyn, for example, describes the scene in Trenton, which lay on the main road to New York. Every day the people would rush to read the newspapers dropped off by the northbound stages. In his letters to Robert Ralston in Wilmington, John Welsh routinely included accounts from the *Federal Gazette*. At first he sent copies of the paper, but in October he arranged with Andrew Brown to start a subscription for Ralston, to be dispatched to Wilmington by post. Even after Ralston's subscription had begun, Welsh continued to cite the newspaper in his letters, once copying an item verbatim. "As you will not have the newspapers till Monday evening," he explained, "I will transcribe a piece out of last evening's." In her diary in late October, Elizabeth Drinker cited the newspaper as her source for the total number dead, and in early November she copied verbatim the *Federal Gazette*'s announcement that the fever was over.[41] The surviving manuscript records suggest that Andrew Brown may have exaggerated little when he said he had learned from people all over the country that they had relied on his newspaper for "the most accurate information" on the fever.[42]

As people turned to newspapers for authoritative information, the authorities moved to gain control of the newspapers, especially the *Federal Gazette*, the only major daily in publication after mid-September.[43] After the first week or so of chaos and panic, the public officials and institutional leaders of Philadelphia began to reassert their authority. Their major task, of course, was organization—organization of community resources to meet the crisis. But part of their task was communication. Like the people of Philadelphia and the nation, the leadership elite of the city was obsessed with the news. It was obsessed, however, not with reading the news, but with shaping it.

The first efforts to control the flow of news involved the mayor, Matthew Clarkson, and the prestigious College of Physicians of Philadelphia. In 1793, Philadelphia was home to the best medical minds in America, and the College of Physicians was their temple. Here gathered the leading doctors of the new republic to honor and advance medical science and themselves.[44] Naturally, the desperate mayor turned to the College for help in confronting the looming catastrophe. The fellows of the College met on 25 August to draft a list of recommendations to be published in the newspapers. Dr. Rush wrote the report, passed it along to the mayor, and two days later it appeared in print.[45]

In the weeks after 27 August, Mayor Clarkson (and other public officials) peppered the papers with official information. These communiqués included a variety of public orders (on sanitation, ship inspections, etc.) as well as announcements of "authenticated" fever news. The news ranged from notices of the work of organizations to official statements on the death toll of the week—the latter aimed at dispelling the extravagant rumors of wholesale slaughter. At times, the mayor used the press to squelch a specific rumor, such as an erroneous report that the fever had infected the city jail. These pieces were printed verbatim, usually in the form of signed letters, and often with the tag line: "The printers of newspapers in the city are requested to insert the above."[46]

On 14 September, Mayor Clarkson called together an extraordinary citizens' committee to supervise the city's response to the epidemic. This committee of volunteers, with Clarkson presiding, stood as virtually the only public authority in Philadelphia at the height of the fever. "The Committee," as it was called, quickly gained a reputation for practicality, efficiency, and quiet heroism. The tasks of the Committee included distribution of provisions to the poor, care of impoverished orphans, and supervision of a makeshift charity hospital located at Bush Hill, the country seat of a local gentle-man.[47] The distribution of tangible services to the sick and poor was the Committee's top priority. But distribution of information to the newspapers ranked high as well. Again and again, in its official minutes, the Committee directed its secretary "to hand to the printer of the *Federal Gazette* for publica-tion" a certain report or "to cause the following communication to be printed for the information of our fellow citizens."[48]

An early aim of these official reports was to quash the rumors that admis-sion to Bush Hill was a death sentence. One reader wrote to the *Federal Gazette* in early September to complain about the lack of reliable information about Bush Hill. "We ought at least to have been informed by public authenticity, how it is attended," he said. "This will have at least one wholesome effect—it will stop the gossiping reports of idle people." The Committee was soon able to reply, in official reports to the newspaper, that conditions at Bush Hill were im-proving daily. The accommodations were now sanitary, the doctors and nurses competent, and the course of treatment salubrious.[49] In early October, the Com-mittee turned to the newspaper to attack rumors that all the outlying towns were hostile and unsympathetic to Philadelphia's plight. The Committee or-dered dozens of letters published that told of public sympathy and relief cam-paigns in other cities and states. And, at long last, the Committee used the newspaper in late October to announce officially the end of the epidemic.[50]

Though the College of Physicians faded early in the epidemic as an institu-tional voice of authority, individual doctors continued to count the dissemina-tion of information among their major duties. Indeed, it sometimes seemed as if the newspaper article was the chief instrument of medical practice in Philadel-phia in 1793. The doctors wrote newspaper articles for two somewhat separate reasons: to serve the public and to establish the authority of a particular mode of treatment. In the doctors' minds, of course, these reasons were identical.

Among the physicians of Philadelphia, the leading newspaper writer was Benjamin Rush. Though Rush had composed the College of Physicians' ini-tial report on the fever, he soon grew dissatisfied with his colleagues' timidity in treating it. In early September, Rush discovered his own cure for the yel-low fever: heroic purging and copious bleeding. With powerful doses of calomel (a mercury compound) and liberal use of the lancet, Rush believed the fever could be weakened and defeated.[51] Instantly, he turned to the press to publicize his discovery. The first announcement of "Dr. Rush's Directions for Curing and Preventing the Yellow Fever" appeared in the *Federal Gazette* on 11 September. From that day forth, a day rarely passed without some refer-ence in the newspaper to Dr. Benjamin Rush.

Rush used the newspaper partly to save time. After tending to upwards of one hundred patients in a day, Rush spent his evenings answering letters from anxious doctors in the countryside, and writing to his family. He could neither see enough patients nor answer enough mail to meet the demands laid upon him. Indeed, he said that merely reading all the letters was nearly beyond his endurance. So, he prescribed in print. At the height of the fever, he wrote to his wife:

> To save the trouble of writing answers to each of them, I have this evening composed a short account of the origin, symptoms, and treatment of the disease which I shall address to Dr. Rodgers of New York in the form of a letter and publish in Mr. Brown's paper. My postage for letters frequently amounts to 7/6 a day.[52]

But for Rush medical practice via newspaper made political as well as practical sense, for Rush believed (or so he said) in a republican medicine. Virulent diseases such as the yellow fever were actually quite simple enough for anyone to understand.[53] His aim, therefore, was "to teach the people to cure themselves by my publications in the newspapers." Cure themselves. This was a recurrent theme in the writings of this life-long American patriot and republican, who could declare with conviction that "the people rule here in medicine as well as government."[54] In other words, Dr. Rush believed that the yellow fever could be cured by purging, bleeding, and reading the newspaper.

Yet his faith in the people was not equal to his faith in himself. When people disparaged his heroic cures, he pressed on with them, because he knew that he was right, that truth was on his side. And his truth was derived from logic and theory, more than from experimental or empirical (or, one might well add, republican) practice. Though he daily worked himself to exhaustion among the sick and dying, his true research was done in his study, not in the streets and sickrooms of Philadelphia. "I applied myself with fresh ardor to the investigation of the disease before me," he wrote. "I ransacked my library, and pored over every book that treated of the yellow fever."[55] Certainly, Rush believed that he was an experimentalist. He believed that he could see the good results in practice. But, fundamentally, Rush's cure was based on abstract principle and wishful thinking, not on systematic observation and experiment. Thus, much of his newspaper writing during the fever consisted of the quotation of authoritative medical sources.[56]

Most of Rush's colleagues abhorred virtually all of his ideas about the epidemic, except his belief in the power and utility of the press. Like Rush, they turned to the newspapers to disseminate their theories and to establish their authority. On the same day that Rush's directions for purging and bleeding appeared in the *Federal Gazette*, Dr. Adam Kuhn published a long piece denouncing emetics and laxatives and favoring mild teas and barks. The next day Rush published a rejoinder. And the flood-gates were opened.[57] Almost daily thereafter the *Federal Gazette* was heavily laden with the writings of the physicians of Philadelphia. Most claimed public service and service to the truth as their only motives. In a typical opening, Dr. Thomas Ruston wrote:

> At a time when the public mind is so much agitated by the prevalence of a very alarming disease, . . . it becomes the duty of every good citizen to step forward, and to contribute his mite, not only to quiet those alarms, but if possible to assist in removing the cause.[58]

Though they spoke of quieting the public alarm, the doctors were more concerned about the victory of their theories. The rancor and hostility rose with the death toll. And the entire controversy was played out in the newspaper. In support of Dr. Kuhn, Dr. William Currie wrote that Rush's treatment "cannot fail of being certain death. . . . It is time the veil should be withdrawn from your eyes, my fellow citizens!" In support of Dr. Rush, Dr. Robert Annan denounced Currie's "bold ignorance" and declared that such a man "is not fit to be reasoned with."[59] Meanwhile, Rush brooded and fulminated:

> They have confederated against me in the most cruel manner and are propagating calumnies against me in every part of the city. Dr. Currie (my old friend) is now the weak instrument of their malice and prejudices. If I outlive the present calamity, I know not when I shall be safe from their persecutions. Never did I before witness such a mass of ignorance and wickedness as our profession has exhibited in the course of the present calamity.[60]

Rush believed that the publications of his enemies were killing people by the hundreds. "I was contending," he wrote years later, "with the most criminal ignorance, and the object of the contest was the preservation of a city."[61]

Many readers were dismayed by the doctors' newspaper war. Ebenezer Hazard expressed a sentiment that is not uncommon in the surviving manuscript letters: "Our physicians differ in sentiment both about the nature of the disorder and the mode of treating it, and have added to the general distress by publishing their contradictory opinions in the newspapers."[62] Some readers were unhappy enough to publish their complaints. "A Citizen" wrote to the *Federal Gazette*:

> From such a contrariety of sentiments, what are we to conclude, or how shall we act? It would be well if those gentlemen would consider the perturbation, the extreme anxiety and distress, with which those publications have filled the minds of their fellow citizens.[63]

In a few of the letters, the perturbation was palpable. One exasperated reader wrote to Andrew Brown:

For God's sake!—for the sake of those who daily wait for the publication of the *Federal Gazette*, with anxiety! and for your own sake! let your readers be no more pestered with disputes about a doctrine, which hath been a bone of contention for a couple of centuries.[64]

In short, both elite and regular readers turned to the newspaper in the terrible autumn of 1793 for authoritative news, for "authentic intelligence." But what they sometimes found were rumors, contradictions, and arcane ideological disputes among the doctors. This confusion of authority worried the would-be authorities very much. But what could be done about it? One approach would be to make the printed word more formally and systematically the voice of authority. This is precisely what Mathew Carey proposed to city health officials the next autumn, when it appeared that the fever would visit Philadelphia once again. He reminded them of the terror that was spread by false reports and contradictory news in 1793. He then added:

The remedy is obvious. Let the genuine truth be made known. Let such a respectable body of men as you are—a body in whom not only our own citizens, but those of the other states, will place implicit reliance—publish daily, or otherwise as you may judge proper, a faithful, unvarnished state of the business.[65]

But was a faithful, unvarnished report all that mattered? Was "authentic intelligence" all that readers expected from their newspaper in the throes of a crisis like the yellow fever? The evidence suggests that the newspaper played for its readers a much richer and more complicated role than this.

"EVERY OBSERVATION"

Mr. Brown,

As every observation on the present prevailing disorder, founded on fact, may have its use, you will please publish the following.[66]

The man who wrote that sentence in a letter to the *Federal Gazette* seems to have been neither a public official nor a doctor. He was merely a citizen of Philadelphia and a reader of the newspaper. He caught the fever; he recovered; and now he wanted to share his experience and his remedy with others. His personal story was a bit rambling, but his cure was simple: molasses. Over the three-day course of the fever he took about two quarts of molasses, which produced, among other things, "very great discharges of wind, which the disorder seems to generate in great quantities in the stomach, which wind is perhaps the fatal instrument of destruction." He ended his letter with the obvious recommendation: "Perhaps the daily use of molasses in its common form, or mixed with water, might at this time be beneficial."

The sharing of personal experiences and folk remedies was just one of several uses that common readers made of the newspaper, uses that ranged far beyond the domain of official pronouncements and authenticated information. Readers also came to the newspaper to make suggestions to public officials, to thank people, to explain the religious meaning of the fever, to defend the civic honor of Philadelphia, and to try to disarm the terror with humor and satire. Each of these uses suggests the desire—perhaps the compelling need—of readers to participate in the community's response to the epidemic by participating in the newspaper.

Throughout the epidemic, but especially in the early weeks before the doctors' pens were fully mobilized, the newspapers published dozens of letters from readers recommending a fascinating variety of folk cures and preventatives. On the same day that the molasses man told his story, another reader proclaimed "earth bathing" as the "universal remedy." Others liked earth as well. One reader recommended covering sickroom floors with fresh earth; another suggested burying the linens of death beds in the ground for three days. Still other correspondents prescribed smoke, vinegar, camphor, tar, garlic, rue, wormwood, lavender, and pennyroyal. Some proposed cleanliness, temperance, and cheerfulness.[67] And so on. In a rare commercial endorsement, one reader said he had tried "quack medicines and nostrums of every kind," but "candor must acknowledge that none has yet appeared to compare with Delany's Aromatic Distilled Vinegar."[68]

Besides recommending cures, these letters often included personal narratives, and they were frequently prefaced by statements asserting every citizen's right and duty to contribute information to the public through the press. For example, the earth-bather declared that "every method of prevention and cure for diseases in general, and for this present epidemic in particular, ought to be made known to the public." Another said, "It behooves every friend of humanity, who may possess the smallest knowledge of any means whereby the present unhappy malady may be checked, or prevented from spreading, to publish such useful hints as may have this tendency." All seemed to agree with "A Friend to the Public," who admitted that his cure (tobacco smoke) may not work, but surely "a trial cannot be amiss in this time of public calamity."[69]

Some readers made suggestions to public officials through the newspapers. One letter writer argued that fires in the streets were useless and that the city should ban them. Several days later Mayor Clarkson did just that. Citizens wrote to urge the city to appoint more police guards and to see to it that people who leave town leave their fire buckets in a public place. The city followed up on those suggestions, too. Others offered advice to the Committee. Of course, not all of the advice was equally well taken. One reader wrote that the West Indians had discovered that nothing stops yellow fever better than the firing of cannon. He added that the people of Philadelphia "would cheerfully pay the expense of the powder, and I am sure that General Proctor would with pleasure attend the firing." This nostrum proved instantly unpalatable. Mayor Clarkson quickly moved to ban the shooting of guns in the streets of the city—via a notice in the newspaper, of course.[70]

Readers also used the newspaper to make public their thankfulness. Some offered words of general thanksgiving to the mayor, the Committee, the ministers, and the doctors ("those intrepid sons of Galen") who served the city faithfully and selflessly. "Blessed be the corporation," one writer declared, "for their attention to whatever concerns the health of our city." Others thanked specific people, often their doctors or pastors. Like most letters in the paper, these were usually unsigned. Of those that were signed, the writers ranged from Secretary of the Treasury Alexander Hamilton to lumber merchant James Corkrin to baker Frederick Fraley.[71] Along with their praise and thanks, several letters carried notes of censure for doctors and ministers who forsook their public duties and fled the city. One reader even suggested that the worthy and unworthy be identified publicly—in the newspaper.[72]

For the doctors, the mayor, and the Committee, the fever was purely a problem of medicine and public health. But for many readers of the newspaper, the epidemic was an event charged with religious and moral meaning. And they used the newspaper to proclaim this belief. "I have waited with longing expectation," a reader wrote, "in hopes that some able and well-disposed persons would take up their pen, and state their ideas of the real causes of the chastisements of the inhabitants of this city." What were the real causes? "Pride, speculation, and ambition ... Playhouses, circus, palaces, carriages, and costly edifices." Sounding a call that would become commonplace, another correspondent declared: "Instead of fleeing from the city during the present visitation of Divine Providence, the inhabitants should give themselves time to reflect, and humble themselves under JEHOVAH's awful rod."[73] Religious people did not deny the natural origin of the disease, but they saw behind nature the agency of God; and, thus, they saw within the fever a divine commentary on the corruption of community life in Philadelphia.[74]

On the other hand, more readers were defenders than critics of Philadelphia. As news of the epidemic spread, other cities and towns acted, sometimes rather harshly, to repel the refugees as well as the disease itself. These quarantine actions, publicized in the newspapers, aroused a spirit of community pride and solidarity in the readers of the *Federal Gazette*.[75] One blasted the "cruelty and selfishness" of these towns: "Ye unfeeling savages! Ye monsters in the shape of men! 'How can you hope for mercy rendering none?'" Another conceded the need to control the spread of the fever, but asked, "Why no expression illustrative of your tender feelings? Are we not your brothers?" Still others urged Philadelphians to come together as a community in defiance of the censorious outside world. "Let New York, Trenton, and Baltimore resolve and re-resolve that we may all perish together," one reader exclaimed; "we are resolving under Providence to live, in spite of all their cruel resolves." Another summed up the feeling quite nicely: "Let us, my fellow citizens, bear in mind that we are members of one common family; that, as such, we ought by no means to desert one another in the moment of our suffering."[76]

When the suffering was most intense, some readers of the *Federal Gazette* tried to break the tension with humor and satire. In late September and early October, Brown published two satiric dialogues sent in by readers. One of them, which tells the story of a Philadelphia man's cold reception in New Jersey, spoofs both the hostility of the surrounding countryside and the doctors' controversy over cures. A farmer greets the man with a pitchfork. "Ho!—Who are you, you yellow-fever looking fellow, and what business have you out of your city?" The man replies that he is perfectly healthy. The farmer is unconvinced. "Why, sir, your breath is pestilence. . . . You are a moving mass of putridity, corruption, plague, poison, and putrefaction." When the farmer refuses to let him stay the night, the Philadelphian asks to buy some meat. "Beef for a man in your situation!—You are, beyond all doubt, raving mad, and light-headed. If you were in your right senses, you would rather ask for tartar-emetic, jalaps, purges, collery morbus, ippecaanha, doses of Spanish flies, and cartloads of drugs, physics, and medicines of every denomination and description."[77]

The second dialogue also takes place in New Jersey, this time between two farmers, with George telling William of his harrowing trip into the city. Before crossing the Delaware, George had stopped up all his bodily orifices—the two lower ones with a cork and a stout leather string, his ears and nose with putty, and his mouth with a handkerchief. As he crossed the river, he could see that the city was as yellow as a pumpkin patch. In town, people were dropping dead in the street, left and right. Yet he made it to the market and sold his eggs for four shillings and his butter for five shillings ninepence. He would have gotten more, he said, but he couldn't haggle properly through his gag. William was impressed by the scenes of death and devastation, but more impressed by the high prices. Tomorrow, he said, he would go to Philadelphia.[78]

ISOLATION AND COMMUNICATION

Instead of equipages and a throng of passengers, the voice of levity and glee, which I had formerly observed, and which the mildness of the season would, at other times, have produced, I found nothing but a dreary solitude.[79]

34

When Charles Brockden Brown's fictional hero Arthur Mervyn enters Philadelphia during the 1793 epidemic, he is struck most forcefully by the eerie isolation that the fever has fastened upon the inhabitants of the city. Mervyn comes into town from the west along Market Street at nightfall:

> The market-place, and each side of this magnificent avenue, were illuminated, as before, by lamps; but between the verge of the Schuylkill and the heart of the city I met not more than a dozen figures; and these were ghost-like, wrapped in cloaks, from behind which they cast upon me glances of wonder and suspicion, and, as I approached, changed their course, to avoid touching me. . . . I cast a look upon the houses, which I recollected to have formerly been, at this hour, brilliant with lights, resounding with lively voices, and thronged with busy faces. Now they were closed, above and below; dark, and without tokens of being inhabited. From the upper windows of some, a gleam sometimes fell upon the pavement I was traversing, and showed that their tenants had not fled, but were secluded or disabled.[80]

This theme of isolation runs through all of the fever narratives. Jacob Hiltzheimer wrote in his diary in mid-September that "very few people walk the streets, and if it is known to your friends that any of your family are sick they avoid you." Isaac Heston wrote to his brother that "those who have not removed are afraid to see anybody, even their nearest friends, and keep themselves close confined in their houses, and this city never wore so gloomy an aspect before." Many years later, Robert Simpson recalled the same doleful scene:

> It was indeed melancholy to walk the streets, which were completely deserted, except by carts having bells attached to the horses heads, on hearing which the dead bodies were put outside on the pavement and placed in the carts by the negroes, who conveyed their charge to the first grave yard, when they returned for another load.[81]

With thousands dying, thousands fleeing, and thousands cowering from the supposed contagion, isolation was inevitable. Yet some people argued that there wasn't isolation enough, and that isolation should be imposed upon the city by law as well as by choice. The College of Physicians had recommended that the sick be avoided, and several letters in the *Federal Gazette* in the weeks following urged city officials to enforce this recommendation. One letter writer called for the suspension of all social contact—business meetings, church services, sick calls, funerals. Another agreed that there was too much contact, too much talking. All social intercourse should cease, he said, for "the general anxiety for information about the sick has been the speedy means of spreading death and terror around us."[82] And, of course, the newspapers were criticized for spreading fear and rumor.

In spite of hazard, warning, and threat, however, the "anxiety for information" overwhelmed the fear of death. Many people simply would not stop visiting, would not stop talking, would not stop communicating. Throughout the epidemic, church services and Quaker meetings continued, even flourished, despite strong sentiment against them. Nervous parishioners smoked their churches and doused themselves with vinegar, but still they came together.[83] And beyond these face-to-face congregations of people, the communication was perhaps even more intense. Day after day, the letters flowed and the newspapers circulated. In his account of the fever, Dr. Rush made a small but significant point. He said that no one ever believed that the disease could be transmitted by paper; thus, people were able to maintain the bonds of written and printed communication.[84] And these bonds—the bonds of communication—were important, perhaps more important than all the nostrums the good doctors could devise.

In a sense, the isolation imposed by the yellow fever and the hunger for communication that it generated are only extrapolations, intensifications of the ordinary impact of urban life on the inhabitants of the modern city. In cities, people are thrust together, yet separated; they are neighbors, yet strangers. And much of urban institutional life might be seen as an effort to bridge these gaps. Central to this effort, as I have tried to show, has been reading the newspaper. Newspapers, of course, do not bring everyone in the city together. Like other urban institutions, they have often been instruments of division as well as connection. But in America, where literacy rates were high, they have sometimes served as important construction sites for the building of new forms of public community in the modern, impersonal metropolis.[85]

In 1791, two years before the yellow fever crisis, Andrew Brown described the virtue of newspaper reading as sympathy in solitude. That phrase, I think, begins to capture the special role of the newspaper (and perhaps of reading in general) in modern community life. People can be separated, yet in communion. But the phrase suggests a more passive reader than the readers I followed through the yellow fever epidemic of 1793. These readers were active. With notes, letters, discussions, arguments, prayers, and meditations—in the newspaper and out of it—they replenished the texts of public discourse. For these readers, newspaper readership was a form of active citizenship, a way to participate in the on-going conversation of their community.[86]

NOTES

1. *Federal Gazette*, 9 September 1793. All newspapers cited in this chapter were published in Philadelphia. The *Federal Gazette* was the only one to remain in business

throughout the yellow fever epidemic of 1793. I have standardized eighteenth-century spelling in all citations.

2. On the effort to build a history of reading—i.e., to move the historical study of literacy toward the study of actual readers—see Carl F. Kaestle et al., *Literacy in the United States: Readers and Reading since 1880* (New Haven: Yale University Press, 1991), chapters 1 and 2; David D. Hall, "Readers and Reading in America: Historical and Critical Perspectives," *Proceedings of the American Antiquarian Society*, 103 (1993): 337–357; Robert Darnton, "First Steps Toward a History of Reading," in Darnton, *The Kiss of Lamourette: Reflections in Cultural History* (New York: W.W. Norton, 1990); and Jonathan Rose, "Rereading the English Common Reader: A Preface to a History of Audiences," *Journal of the History of Ideas*, 53 (1992): 47–70.

3. Mathew Carey, *A Short Account of the Malignant Fever, lately Prevalent in Philadelphia*, 4th ed. (Philadelphia: Mathew Carey, 1794), p. 22. General accounts of the 1793 yellow fever include John Harvey Powell, *Bring Out Your Dead: The Great Plague of Yellow Fever in Philadelphia in 1793* (Philadelphia: University of Pennsylvania Press, 1949); Charles-Edward A. Winslow, *The Conquest of Epidemic Disease* (Princeton, N.J.: Princeton University Press, 1943), chapter 11; Martin S. Pernick, "Politics, Parties, and Pestilence: Epidemic Yellow Fever in Philadelphia and the Rise of the First Party System," *William and Mary Quarterly*, 3rd ser., 29 (1972): 559–86 [reprinted in this volume]; Richard G. Miller, "The Federal City, 1783–1800," in *Philadelphia: A 300-Year History*, ed. Russell F. Weigley (New York: W.W. Norton, 1982); and Eve Kornfeld, "Crisis in the Capital: The Cultural Significance of Philadelphia's Great Yellow Fever Epidemic," *Pennsylvania History* 51 (1984): 189–205. Broader medical/social histories of the disease include William Coleman, *Yellow Fever in the North: The Methods of Early Epidemiology* (Madison: University of Wisconsin Press, 1987); Margaret Humphreys, *Yellow Fever and the South* (New Brunswick, N.J.: Rutgers University Press, 1992); James C. Riley, *The Eighteenth-Century Campaign to Avoid Disease* (New York: St. Martin's Press, 1987); and K. David Patterson, "Yellow Fever Epidemics and Mortality in the United States, 1693–1905," *Social Science and Medicine* 34 (1992): 855–865.

4. My understanding of reader communities has been aided by Janice Radway, "Interpretive Communities and Variable Literacies: The Functions of Romance Reading," *Daedalus* 113 (Summer, 1984): 49–73; Cathy N. Davidson, *Revolution and the Word: The Rise of the Novel in America* (New York: Oxford University Press, 1986), chapter 1; Norman N. Holland, *The Critical I* (New York: Columbia University Press, 1992); Stanley Fish, *Is There a Text in This Class?: The Authority of Interpretive Communities* (Cambridge: Harvard University Press, 1980); and the essays in *Reader-Response Criticism: From Formalism to Post-Structuralism*, ed. Jane P. Tompkins (Baltimore: Johns Hopkins University Press, 1980).

5. Of course, many residents of Philadelphia, including slaves and the transient poor, were excluded from this reader community because they could not read, or could not read English. Yet even illiterates were sometimes part of oral communities that were linked through literates to the print culture of the city.

6. *Federal Gazette*, 6 December 1791.

7. Sam Bass Warner, *The Private City: Philadelphia in Three Periods of Its Growth* (Philadelphia: University of Pennsylvania Press, 1968), p. 11.

8. Benjamin Davies, *Some Account of the City of Philadelphia* (Philadelphia: Richard Folwell, 1794), pp. 16–18, 80. See also Gary B. Nash and Billy G. Smith, "The Population of Eighteenth-Century Philadelphia," *Pennsylvania Magazine of History and Biography* 99 (1975): 362–68; Miller, "The Federal City"; and Susan E. Klepp, *Philadelphia in Transition: A Demographic History of the City and Its Occupational Groups, 1720–1830* (New York: Garland Press, 1989).

9. Richard G. Miller, *Philadelphia—The Federalist City: A Study of Urban Politics, 1789–1801* (Port Washington, N.Y.: Kennikat Press, 1976), pp. 5–6; John K. Alexander, *Render Them Submissive: Responses to Poverty in Philadelphia, 1760–1800* (Amherst: University of Massachusetts Press, 1980), p. 12; Billy G. Smith, *The "Lower Sort": Philadelphia's Laboring People, 1750–1800* (Ithaca: Cornell University Press, 1990), chapters 3 and 4; Billy G. Smith, "Inequality in Late Colonial Philadelphia: A Note on Its Nature and Growth," *William and Mary Quarterly*, 3rd ser., 41 (1984): 629–45; Sharon V. Salinger, "Artisans, Journeymen, and the Transformation of Labor in Late-Eighteenth-Century Philadelphia," *William and Mary Quarterly*, 3rd ser., 40 (1983): 62–84.

10. Miller, *Philadelphia*, pp. 4 (quotation), 6–8.

11. Gary B. Nash, "The Social Evolution of Preindustrial American Cities, 1700–1820: Reflections and New Directions," *Journal of Urban History* 13 (1987): 119, 133.

12. Ibid., p. 119; Gary B. Nash, *Forging Freedom: The Formation of Philadelphia's Black Community, 1720–1840* (Cambridge: Harvard University Press, 1988). See also Thomas Bender, *Community and Social Change in America* (New Brunswick, N.J.: Rutgers University Press, 1978), chapters 1 and 2.

13. Like Michael Warner, I am interested in how publication was related to public life in the late eighteenth century. While Warner explores the republican discourse itself, I'm concerned with how ordinary readers participated in it. See Warner, *The Letters of the Republic: Publication and the Public Sphere in Eighteenth-Century America* (Cambridge: Harvard University Press, 1990). Recent studies of actual readers in this era include Richard D. Brown, *Knowledge Is Power: The Diffusion of Information in Early America, 1700–1865* (New York: Oxford University Press, 1989); and William J. Gilmore, *Reading Becomes a Necessity of Life: Material and Cultural Life in Rural New England* (Knoxville: University of Tennessee Press, 1989).

14. Warner, *Private City*, p. 20. See also Carl Bridenbaugh, "The Press and the Book in Eighteenth-Century Philadelphia," *Pennsylvania Magazine of History and Biography* 65 (1941): 1–30; Edwin Wolf II, *The Book Culture of a Colonial City: Philadelphia Books, Bookmen, and Booksellers* (New York: Oxford University Press, 1988).

15. Davies, *Some Account*, p. 83; William F. Steirer, Jr., "Philadelphia Newspapers: Years of Revolution and Transition, 1764–1794" (Ph.D. diss., University of Pennsylvania, 1972), pp. 228–29, 310, 347.

16. "The Newspaper," in the *Pennsylvania Packet*, 22 September 1784.

17. Samuel Magaw, *A Discourse Occasioned by the Mournful Catastrophe, through Fire, Which Destroyed Mr. Andrew Brown, his Wife, and Three Children* (Philadelphia: Ormrod & Conrad, 1797), n.p.; "An Essay on the Utility of Newspapers" and "To

the Public," in the *Philadelphia Gazette*, 1 January 1794. Brown changed the name of the *Federal Gazette* to the *Philadelphia Gazette* in 1794 to disassociate it from the emerging Federalist Party.

18. *Federal Gazette*, 1 October 1788. Brown reaffirmed this booster role in his inaugural issue of the *Philadelphia Gazette*, 1 January 1794.

19. *Federal Gazette*, 29 October 1788, 1 October 1793, and 25 November 1793.

20. Ibid., 6 December 1791. See also Steirer, "Philadelphia Newspapers," p. 80; and Dwight L. Teeter, Jr., "John Dunlap: The Political Economy of a Printer's Success," *Journalism Quarterly* 52 (1975): 3–8, 55.

21. *Federal Gazette*, 26 October 1793; *Philadelphia Gazette*, 1 January 1794.

22. Robert Simpson, Letterbook, 1788–1807, Historical Society of Pennsylvania; Robert Simpson, "Narrative of a Scottish Adventurer," *Journal of the Presbyterian Historical Society* 27 (1949): 48–49. Simpson's wish came true less than three years later. Brown and his family were killed in a house fire. See *American Daily Advertiser*, 7 February 1797; and Magaw, *A Discourse*.

23. Simpson, Letterbook; Powell, *Bring Out Your Dead*, pp. 141–42, 256. Most contemporary accounts of the epidemic mention the importance of the newspapers, especially the *Federal Gazette*. I found only one disparaging comment on the utility of the newspaper in the crisis. It appeared in Benjamin Franklin Bache's paper—in an effort after the epidemic to justify to his readers his own decision to suspend publication. See *General Advertiser*, 25 November 1793.

24. *Federal Gazette*, 26 October 1793.

25. John Fenno to Joseph Ward, 8 October 1793, in "Letters of John Fenno and John Ward Fenno, 1779–1800; Part 2, 1792–1800," ed. John B. Hench, *Proceedings of the American Antiquarian Society* 91 (1980): 177. The original letters are in the Joseph Ward Collection, Chicago Historical Society.

26. Benjamin Rush to Julia Rush, 25 September 1793, in *Letters of Benjamin Rush*, ed. L.H. Butterfield, 2 vols. (Princeton, N.J.: Princeton University Press, 1951), 2: 640. See also Nathan G. Goodman, *Benjamin Rush: Physician and Citizen, 1746–1813* (Philadelphia: University of Pennsylvania Press, 1934), pp. 170–71; Benjamin Rush, *An Enquiry into the Origin of the Late Epidemic Fever in Philadelphia* (Philadelphia: Mathew Carey, 1793); Rush, *An Account of the Bilious Remitting Yellow Fever, as it Appeared in the City of Philadelphia, in the Year 1793* (Philadelphia: Thomas Dobson, 1794), pp. 14–15.

27. Rush to Julia Rush, 25, 27, 29 August 1793, in *Letters of Benjamin Rush*, 2: 640–45; William Currie, *A Treatise on the Synochus Icteroides, or Yellow Fever, as It Lately Appeared in the City of Philadelphia* (Philadelphia: Thomas Dobson, 1794), p. 3; *Minutes of the Proceedings of the Committee, Appointed on the 14th September, 1793, . . . To Attend to and Alleviate the Sufferings of the Afflicted with the Malignant Fever* (Philadelphia: City of Philadelphia, 1848), p. 137. These minutes were originally printed in 1794 by R. Aitken of Philadelphia. Evans lists thirty-nine titles dealing with the yellow fever in his 1793 and 1794 volumes. See Charles Evans, *American Bibliography* (New York: Peter Smith, 1941). The most widely circulated contemporary account was Carey, *Short Account*. For mortality rates, see Tom W. Smith, "The Dawn of the Urban-Industrial Age: The Social Structure of Philadelphia, 1790–1830" (Ph.D. diss., University of Chicago, 1980), pp. 89–90 and passim.

28. Carey, *Short Account*, p. 23. See also Sally F. Griffith's essay in this volume.
29. Ibid., p. 25. The heroic organizational response to the fever is a common theme in contemporary accounts. For example, see David Nassy, *Observations on the Cause, Nature, and Treatment of the Epidemic Disorder Prevalent in Philadelphia* (Philadelphia: Parker & Co., 1793), pp. 43–44; Jean Deveze, *An Enquiry into and Observations upon the Causes and Effects of the Epidemic Disease which Raged in Philadelphia* (Philadelphia: Pierre Parent, 1794), passim.; A[bsalom] J[ones] and R[ichard] A[llen], *A Narrative of the Proceedings of the Black People, during the Late Awful Calamity in Philadelphia* (Philadelphia: William Woodward, 1794), p. 10; James Hardie, *The Philadelphia Directory and Register*, 2nd ed. (Philadelphia: Jacob Johnson, 1794), p. 219; *Poulson's Town and Country Almanac, for the Year of Our Lord 1795* (Philadelphia: Zachariah Poulson, 1794); *Banneker's Almanac for the Year 1795* (Philadelphia: William Young, 1794).
30. Samuel Stearns, *An Account of the Terrible Effects of the Pestilential Infection in the City of Philadelphia* (Providence, R.I.: William Child, 1793), pp. 5–6.
31. Carey, *Short Account*, p. 45.
32. This generalization is based upon a fairly extensive reading of published letters and diaries as well as manuscript collections in Philadelphia libraries: The Library Company, the Historical Society of Pennsylvania, the American Philosophical Society, and the College of Physicians of Philadelphia.
33. Carey, *Short Account*, pp. 45–47; Deveze, *An Enquiry*, pp. 10–12; Nassy, *Observations*, p. 9; Joshua Cresson, *Meditations Written during the Prevalence of the Yellow Fever in the City of Philadelphia in the Year 1793* (London: W. Phillips, 1803), p. 7. As terrifying rumors spread from Philadelphia, many outlying communities took steps—sometimes violent steps—to turn fleeing Philadelphians away. The *Federal Gazette* reported on many of these actions. For example, see *Federal Gazette*, 18, 19 September 1793, and 2 October 1793.
34. For example, see Susanna Dillwyn to William Dillwyn, 29 September 1793, in Susanna Dillwyn Correspondence, Library Company manuscripts, housed in the Historical Society of Pennsylvania. Susanna lived in New Jersey; her father, William, in England. Letters to the newspaper made the same plea, and Brown himself warned "our friends in the country" to be slow to believe the rumors they heard. See *Federal Gazette*, 12 September 1793, and 12 October 1793.
35. John Depeyster to Charles Willson Peale, 2, 10 October 1793, in Sellers Family Papers, American Philosophical Society. This is a common theme in the surviving letters. For example, several people wrote this same sort of letter to Benjamin Rush. See S. Baynton to Rush, 3 October 1793, John Bayard to Rush, 9 September 1793, Jacob Rush to Rush, 10 September 1793, in Benjamin Rush Papers, vols. 35–36, Historical Society of Pennsylvania.
36. William Dillwyn to Susanna Dillwyn, 26 November 1793, Susanna Dillwyn to William Dillwyn, 11 September 1793, in Susanna Dillwyn Correspondence.
37. Mary Eddy Hosack to Catherine Wistar, 1 October 1793, in Bache Family Papers, American Philosophical Society.
38. Isaac Heston, "Letter from a Yellow Fever Victim, Philadelphia, 1793," ed. Edwin B. Bronner, *Pennsylvania Magazine of History and Biography* 86 (1962): 206.

39. *The Diary of Elizabeth Drinker*, ed. Elaine Forman Crane, 3 vols. (Boston: North-eastern University Press, 1991), entries for 26 August 1793, 31 August 1793, and 3 September 1793, 1:496, 498, 500, and passim. The rumor about the blacks is a particularly interesting and sad one. In fact, the free black people of Philadelphia worked hard during the epidemic to demonstrate their courage and their willingness to serve the city. They were maligned, nonetheless. See Nash, *Forging Freedom*, pp. 121–25; Jones and Allen, *A Narrative of the Proceedings of the Black People*; and Phillip Lapsansky's essay in this volume.

40. "Extracts from the Diary of Jacob Hiltzheimer of Philadephia," *Pennsylvania Magazine of History and Biography* 16 (1892): 417, entry for 14 October 1793.

41. Susanna Dillwyn to William Dillwyn, 9 September 1793, in Susanna Dillwyn Correspondence; John Welsh to Robert Ralston, 16, 18 September 1793, 14 October 1793, 2 November 1793, in Miscellaneous Collections, Historical Society of Pennsylvania; *Diary of Elizabeth Drinker*, entries for 24 October 1793, and 3 November 1793, 1:523–524. See also John Fenno to Joseph Ward, 8 October 1793, in "Letters of John Fenno and John Ward Fenno," p. 177; Bronner, "Letter from a Yellow Fever Victim," p. 206; and Samuel Massey to Ann Massey, 15 September 1793, Samuel Massey Letters, College of Physicians of Philadelphia.

42. *Federal Gazette*, 1, 26 October 1793. At least one letter to the editor also mentioned people in the countryside avidly reading the paper. See *Federal Gazette*, 26 September 1793.

43. Dunlap's *American Daily Advertiser* and Benjamin Franklin Bache's *General Advertiser* played active roles in the early days of the epidemic, but they suspended publication 14 September and 25 September, respectively, and did not resume until December. The two famous national party papers, John Fenno's *Gazette of the United States* and Philip Freneau's *National Gazette*, were small non-dailies that had little yellow fever material. They also suspended publication.

44. Kornfeld, "Crisis in the Capital," pp. 190–91. See also Whitfield J. Bell, Jr., *The College of Physicians of Philadelphia: A Bicentennial History* (Canton, Mass.: Science History Publications, 1987), chapter 2.

45. Rush, *An Account*, pp. 21–24; Rush to Julia Rush, 25 August 1793, in *Letters of Benjamin Rush*, 2: 641; *Federal Gazette*, 27 August 1793; *American Daily Advertiser*, 27 August 1793. See also Minutes, 1793, in Records of the College of Physicians (manuscript volumes), vol. 1, in College of Physicians of Philadelphia, passim.

46. *Federal Gazette*, September, 1793, nearly every day. An example of an official death toll announcement appeared 7 September. The jail item appeared 19 September.

47. Most contemporary accounts praise the work of the Committee. For example, see *Federal Gazette*, 22 November 1793; *Banneker's Almanac*; Nassy, *Observations*, p. 45; Deveze, *An Enquiry*, passim. Deveze, a French West Indian, was the head doctor at Bush Hill.

48. *Minutes of the Proceedings of the Committee, Appointed on the 14th September, 1793*, pp. 47, 89, 103, and passim. The Committee also urged Carey to write his instant history of the fever. See Mathew Carey, *Address of M. Carey to the Public* (Philadelphia: Mathew Carey, 1794), p. 3.

49. *Federal Gazette*, 11, 17, 19, 23, 27 September 1793, and 2 October 1793.
50. *Federal Gazette*, October, 1793, nearly every day. Letters about relief efforts, sent to the *Federal Gazette* by the Committee, became very common after the middle of the month. On the end of the epidemic, see ibid., 16, 28, 29 October 1793, 1, 4, 14, 22 November 1793.
51. *Federal Gazette*, 12 September 1793. Useful accounts of Dr. Rush's cure are Chris Holmes, "Benjamin Rush and the Yellow Fever," *Bulletin of the History of Medicine* 40 (1966): 246–63; and Mark Workman, "Medical Practice in Philadelphia at the Time of the Yellow Fever Epidemic, 1793," *Pennsylvania Folklife* 27 (1978): 33–39. See also Goodman, *Benjamin Rush*, chapter 8; Carl Binger, *Revolutionary Doctor: Benjamin Rush, 1746–1813* (New York: W.W. Norton, 1966), chapter 11; and essays by Jacquelyn C. Miller and J. Worth Estes in this volume.
52. Rush to Julia Rush, 3 October 1793, and 11 September 1793, in *Letters of Benjamin Rush*, 2: 659, 701. The term "7/6" means seven shillings, six pence. See also *Federal Gazette*, 7 October 1793; and Rush, *An Account*, p. 345. The Rush Papers at the Historical Society of Pennsylvania are filled with letters seeking help and advice.
53. Rush, *An Account*, pp. 329–30; *Federal Gazette*, 15 September 1793; Rush to Julia Rush, 15 September 1793, in *Letters of Benjamin Rush*, 2: 664.
54. Benjamin Rush, *The Autobiography of Benjamin Rush: His "Travels Through Life" together with His Commonplace Book for 1789–1813*, ed. George W. Corner (Princeton, N.J.: Princeton University Press, 1948), p. 97; Rush to Julia Rush, 29 September 1793, in *Letters of Benjamin Rush*, 2: 687.
55. Rush, *An Account*, pp. 12–15, 196; Rush, *Autobiography*, p. 98; Holmes, "Benjamin Rush," p. 254.
56. *Federal Gazette*, 11, 22, 26 October 1793. See also Rush to Julia Rush, 27 October 1793, in *Letters of Benjamin Rush*, 2: 727. Chris Holmes traced the outcome of Rush's cure for some fifty of his patients and found that most lived, despite the fact that purging and bleeding were probably quite harmful treatments. See Holmes, "Benjamin Rush," p. 251.
57. *Federal Gazette*, 11, 12 September 1793. The doctors' dispute is treated at length in Powell, *Bring Out Your Dead*, pp. 206–215.
58. *Federal Gazette*, 23 September 1793. The *Federal Gazette* carried dozens of items from doctors and testimonials on various doctors' cures. The major articles are reprinted in Rush, *An Account*, pp. 207–42. See also Nassy, *Observations*, pp. 11–13.
59. *Federal Gazette*, 17, 21 September 1793.
60. Rush to Julia Rush, 21 September 1793, and 2 October 1793, Rush to Elias Boudinot, 25 September 1793, in *Letters of Benjamin Rush*, 2: 673, 681, 693.
61. Rush, *Autobiography*, pp. 96–97. See also Rush, *An Account*, pp. 308–09.
62. Ebenezer Hazard to Jedediah Morse, 30 September 1793, in Simon Gratz Collection, Historical Society of Pennsylvania; John Welsh to Robert Ralston, 18 September 1793, in Miscellaneous Collections, Historical Society of Pennsylvania; Samuel Massey to Ann Massey, 15 September 1793, Samuel Massey Letters, College of Physicians of Philadelphia; James Pemberton, "A Summary Account of a Contagious Fever which Prevailed in Philadelphia," manuscript journal (1793), p. 1, in College of Physicians of Philadelphia.

63. *Federal Gazette*, 20, 21 September 1793, 3 October 1793. See also Rush, *An Account*, p. 126.

64. *Federal Gazette*, 10 October 1793.

65. Mathew Carey, *Gentlemen, Actuated by a Sincere Regard for the Welfare of Our Common City* . . . (Philadelphia: Mathew Carey, 1794). This is a printed letter sent to the Committee of Health for the City of Philadelphia.

66. *Federal Gazette*, 24 September 1793.

67. *Federal Gazette*, 23, 26, 27, 31 August 1793, 2, 9, 13, 14, 30 September 1793.

68. Ibid., 2 September 1793. Paid ads for Delany's vinegar had already begun to appear. For example, see ibid., 30 August 1793.

69. Ibid., 24, 11, 27, 26 September 1793.

70. Ibid., 24, 29 August 1793, 4, 12, 14 September 1793, 14, 15 October 1793.

71. Ibid., 5, 11 September 1793, 1, 2, 5, 22, 23 October 1793, 5, 22 November 1793.

72. Ibid., 3 October 1793, 11, 22 November 1793.

73. Ibid., 7, 25 September 1793, 3, 5, 15, 16 October 1793, 2, 21 November 1793.

74. J. Henry Helmuth, *A Short Account of the Yellow Fever in Philadelphia for the Reflecting Christian*, trans. Charles Erdmann (Philadelphia: Jones, Hoff, and Derrick, 1794), pp. 10–12. See also Elhanan Winchester, *Wisdom Taught by Man's Mortality; Or the Shortness and Uncertainty of Life . . . Adapted to the Awful Visitation of the City of Philadelphia, by the Yellow Fever, in the Year 1793* (Philadelphia: R. Folwell, 1795).

75. On the defensive actions of other towns, see *Federal Gazette*, 15, 18, 19, 25 September 1793.

76. *Federal Gazette*, 21, 24 September 1793, 2, 5 October 1793. Another illustration of community boosterism was the widespread hostility that arose against Rush when he announced that the disease was not imported but of local origin. Many people construed this as a libel on the climate and quality of life in Philadelphia. See *Federal Gazette*, 18 September 1793; Rush to Julia Rush, 28 October 1793, in *Letters of Benjamin Rush*, 2: 729; and Rush, *An Enquiry*, p. 12.

77. *Federal Gazette*, 28 September 1793.

78. Ibid., 2 October 1793. In humor and satire, the leading paper (before its demise) was Philip Freneau's *National Gazette*. Freneau's paper was thin on fever news, but it carried several of the editor's own satiric barbs and verses. See Powell, *Bring Out Your Dead*, frontispiece and pp. 239–40. See also *National Gazette*, 4, 21 September 1793.

79. Charles Brockden Brown, *Arthur Mervyn, or, Memoirs of the Year 1793*, 2 vols. (Port Washington, N.Y.: Kennikat Press, 1963), 1:140. *Arthur Mervyn* was originally published in two parts in 1799 and 1800.

80. Ibid., p. 140. See also William L. Hedges, "Benjamin Rush, Charles Brockden Brown, and the American Plague Year," *Early American Literature* 7 (1973): 295–311; and Warner, *Letters of the Republic*, chapter 6.

81. "Extracts from the Diary of Jacob Hiltzheimer," p. 417; Bronner, "Letter from a Yellow Fever Victim," p. 206; Simpson, "Narrative," p. 50. See also Samuel Massey to Ann Massey, 12 September 1793, Samuel Massey Letters, College of Physicians of Philadelphia; and Carey, *Short Account*, p. 22. Though many blacks died from the disease, they were thought to be immune; thus, they were recruited as nurses and pallbearers. See Kenneth F. Kiple and Virginia Kiple, "Black Yel-

low Fever Immunities, Innate and Acquired, as Revealed in the American South," *Social Science History* 1 (1977): 419–36. See also essays by Phillip Lapsansky, Sally F. Griffith, and Susan E. Klepp in this volume.

82. *Federal Gazette*, 14, 10 September 1793. See also Carey, *Short Account*, pp. 92–93.

83. Helmuth, *Short Account*, pp. 40–45; Pemberton, "A Summary Account," passim.; Cresson, *Meditations*, passim.; *Federal Gazette*, 5 October 1793.

84. Rush, *An Account*, p. 108. Actually, despite Rush's claim, a few people did fear that the disease could be transmitted by paper, and mail from Philadelphia was occasionally smoked in order to disinfect it.

85. I see the urban newspaper as central to what Michael Warner has called (following Jurgen Habermas) the republican public sphere of eighteenth-century America. See Warner, *Letters of the Republic*, chapter 2. I develop the idea of "public community" more fully in a study of a later period of American urban history. See David Paul Nord, "The Public Community: The Urbanization of Journalism in Chicago," *Journal of Urban History* 11 (1985): 411–41.

86. The verb "replenish" is Norman Holland's, in "Unity Identity Text Self," in *Reader-Response Criticism*, ed. Tompkins, p. 118. Holland, like Stanley Fish, sees the reader as necessarily the key figure in the creation of meaning. See Holland, *The Critical I*, and Fish, *Is There a Text in This Class?* See also the essays in James L. Machor, ed., *Readers in History: Nineteenth-Century American Literature and the Contexts of Response* (Baltimore: Johns Hopkins University Press, 1993).

"A Total Dissolution of the Bonds of Society": Community Death and Regeneration in Mathew Carey's *Short Account of the Malignant Fever*

SALLY F. GRIFFITH

N 14 November 1793, Pennsylvania Governor Thomas Mifflin marked the end of the first major epidemic in the new nation's history by proclaiming 12 December a day of general humiliation, thanksgiving, and prayer. He urged all Pennsylvanians to unite that day "in confessing, with contrite hearts, their manifold sins and transgressions—in acknowledging, with thankful adoration, the mercy and goodness of the Supreme Ruler of the universe," who had delivered the city of Philadelphia from its pestilence, and to pray that henceforth their behavior might be so guided as "to avert from all mankind the evils of war, pestilence and famine."[1] Although Mifflin employed fashionable Deistic terminology in naming God, his proclamation placed the terrifying events of the preceding three months within a traditional religious framework in which such disasters were divine punishment for human sins. As the disease-ravaged city began to awaken from its long nightmare, the process of making sense of what had happened was just beginning.[2]

One day before Governor Mifflin's proclamation, Philadelphia printer and bookseller Mathew Carey published the first edition of *A Short Account of the Malignant Fever, Lately Prevalent in Philadelphia*, an "instant history" of the epidemic "for the information of the public." Disclaiming any attempt at "embellishment or ornament of stile," Carey promised to tell "plain facts in plain language." These statements too reflected long-standing tradition, in this instance of on-the-spot disaster reporting, a mainstay of journalism from its earliest days to the present. Proclaiming their absolute adherence to "plain facts," such disaster stories traded upon the public's fascination with tales of human beings in extremity.[3] An enterprising but struggling publisher, thirty-three-year-old Carey had quickly moved to meet an anticipated demand for authori-

45

A SHORT

ACCOUNT

OF THE

MALIGNANT FEVER,

LATELY PREVALENT IN

PHILADELPHIA:

WITH A STATEMENT OF THE

PROCEEDINGS

THAT TOOK PLACE ON THE SUBJECT IN DIFFERENT
PARTS OF THE

UNITED STATES.

———————

BY MATHEW CAREY.

———————

SECOND EDITION.

═══════

PHILADELPHIA:

PRINTED BY THE AUTHOR.

November 23, 1793.

Title page to Mathew Carey's *Short Account*, 1793. Courtesy of the Library
Company of Philadelphia.

tative news, beginning to write his account in early November as the epidemic waned.[4] The first edition sold out within days, and Carey published a second on 23 November; he quickly dispatched hundreds of copies to his fellow-booksellers in Boston, New York, Annapolis, Baltimore, and points farther south. A third edition followed on 30 November, and a fourth on 16 January 1794; in all, he published and sold over 10,000 copies.[5] It was the first major publishing success in what would prove to be a long and influential career.[6]

Carey's account also began by placing Philadelphia's experience within a providential interpretation, but one with a republican twist. The city's increasing prosperity under the new Constitution, he explained, had led almost inevitably to "luxury" and "extravagance," which prevailed "in a manner very alarming to those who considered how far the virtue, the liberty, and the happiness of a nation depend on its temperance and sober manners."[7] Carey grimly contrasted, in "memento mori" tradition, those heedless days before "the malignant fever, crept in among us, and nipped in the bud the fairest blossoms that imagination could form." The narrative that followed traced the emergence and progress of the hideous plague, illustrated with many similarly pathetic reminders of the possibility of sudden death.[8]

At the same time, paralleling this more traditional, admonitory interpretation, ran a narrative inviting a different, more hopeful interpretation, upon which this essay will focus. Even as he reported on the city's painful experience, Carey fashioned a compelling story about community: the collapse of community under the terrifying burden of the epidemic, and the rebirth of community through the heroic efforts of a small band of public-spirited volunteers drawn from the "middling" ranks of the city.

The final, expanded fourth edition upon which this analysis is based includes seventeen chapters and appendices containing accounts of the great plagues in London and Marseilles, day-by-day charts of burials in the city's various graveyards and of meteorological observations, and an alphabetical list of the names of the dead. This necrology undoubtedly was responsible for many of the sales, as Philadelphians and outsiders alike sought to separate the survivors from the dead. Of the main body of the pamphlet, the second half assembles assorted anecdotes about other cities' treatment of refugees from the epidemic and speculations about the cause and nature of the disorder. But, to later readers, the most compelling part of the account is the core narrative contained in the first eight chapters, tracing in roughly chronological order the progress of the disease and the reactions of Philadelphians to their plight.

In Carey's account, Philadelphians awoke late to the existence of the "disorder" among them, and then responded with "an universal terror." Many of those who could began to flee the city, and the streets were filled with refugees and their belongings. Drained of life, the local economy came to a halt, leaving many workingmen unemployed, "and the streets wore the appearance of gloom and melancholy."[9] Here, as throughout, Carey's vivid descriptions highlighted the central role of emotion and imagination in the experiences of his fellow citizens. Although he had promised to relate "plain facts in plain language," his story depends as much on the subjective as on the ostensibly more objective dimensions of the event. For Carey, who was influenced by the romantic cult of sensibility, one's emotional response to the disaster often determined whether one survived, and, significantly, those who fared best were those who remained closely linked to others.

At first, the city's official institutions and authorities responded as best they could, albeit to little effect. Mayor Matthew Clarkson repeatedly ordered the streets cleaned, and amidst the uncertainty about the precise cause of the fever the College of Physicians of Philadelphia recommended among other things "to avoid all unnecessary intercourse with the infected," and to discontinue such unhelpful practices as burning fires in the streets and tolling bells for the dead. This latter custom had resulted in ringing of bells "almost the whole day, so as to terrify those in health, and drive the sick, as far as the influence of imagination could produce that effect, to their graves." The Guardians of the Poor likewise sought to respond to the growing numbers of indigent victims of the disease; they briefly housed a few at a circus on the edge of the settled portion of the city, but neighbors quickly "threatened to burn or destroy it" if the plague victims were not immediately removed. To establish a hospital out of the city, the Guardians commandeered Bush Hill, the mansion of merchant William Hamilton, and resolved to provide nurses and materials for their care. At that point, however, the committee of Guardians effectively ceased to function as an arm of the city's government, all but three of its members having by this time fled the city. In fact, by early September so many members of established institutions—from the Presidency of the United States on down—had either died or fled the city that "government of every kind was almost wholly vacated."[10]

In the wake of this breakdown of established authority, the city, as Carey depicted it, descended into anarchy. Left to fend for themselves, most people became obsessed with their personal preservation, which ironically left them isolated from human contact. Institutions that had brought people together were closed or deserted—churches, the coffee house, the city library, and three of the four daily papers (here Carey gives a passing nod in a footnote to the contribution of Andrew Brown, publisher of the *Federal Gazette*). Many customary usages of civilized society were abandoned. Even "the most respectable citizens" who died went to the grave unattended and without ritual. The most ordinary forms of human contact were abandoned:

> Acquaintances and friends avoided each other in the streets, and only
> signified their regard by a cold nod. The old custom of shaking hands fell

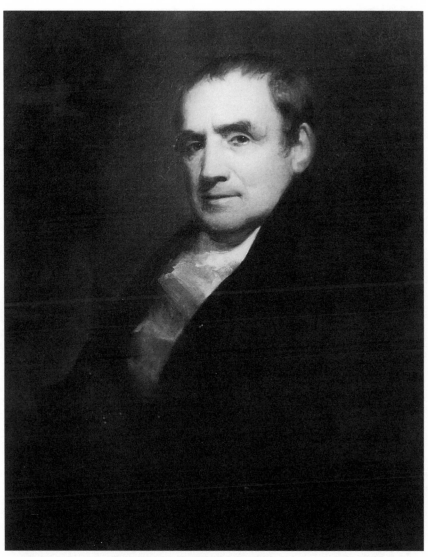

Mathew Carey by John Neagle. Oil on canvas, 1825. Courtesy of the American Philosophical Society.

into such general disuse, that many shrunk back with affright at even the offer of the hand. A person with a crepe, or any appearance of mourning, was shunned like a viper. And many valued themselves highly on the skill and address with which they got to windward of every person whom they met.[11]

The result of this protective isolation was, not surprisingly given Carey's perspective, a state of "general despondency":

When people summoned up resolution to walk abroad, and take the air, the sick cart conveying patients to the hospital, or the hearse carrying the dead to the grave, which were travelling almost the whole day, soon damped their spirits, and plunged them again into despondency.[12]

In such a state of affairs, Carey continued, "we cannot be astonished at the frightful scenes that were acted, which seemed to indicate a total dissolution of the bonds of society in the nearest and dearest connexions." Indeed,

Who, without horror, can reflect on a husband, married perhaps for twenty years, deserting his wife in the last agony—a wife unfeelingly abandoning her husband on his death bed—parents forsaking their only children—children ungratefully flying from their parents, and resigning them to chance, often without an enquiry after their health or safety—masters hurrying off their faithful servants to Bushhill, even on suspicion of the fever, and that at a time, when, like Tartarus, it was open to every visitant, but never returned any—servants abandoning tender and humane masters, who only wanted a little care to restore them to health and usefulness—who, I say, can think of these things without horror? Yet, they were daily exhibited in every quarter of our city; and such was the force of habit, that the parties who were guilty of this cruelty, felt no remorse themselves—nor met with the execration from their fellow-citizens, which such conduct would have excited at any other period. Indeed, at this awful crisis, so much did *self* appear to engross the whole attention of many, that less concern was felt for the loss of a parent, a husband, a wife, or any only child, than, on other occasions, would have been caused by the death of a servant, or even a favourite lap-dog.[13]

I have quoted this passage at length not only because it is the most often-quoted section of his history, but because it represents the heart of his depiction of the epidemic as a sort of social hell, a reversion to a brutal state of nature. Writing about the epidemic in his memoirs precisely thirty years later, Carey himself reprinted this passage to recreate the impact of the disaster.[14] Fear and selfishness reigned, and so consumed Philadelphians that in their search for self-preservation they actually increased their suffering and likelihood of death. Carey recounts episode after episode in which people were left to die untended, when proper care could have preserved them, or in which callous relatives cast out afflicted spouses, only to succumb themselves in turn. An observation in one of the later chapters expanded upon this point. On the one hand, Carey estimated that half to one-third of those who died could have been saved with sufficient attention: "Almost all the remarkable cases of recovery are to be ascribed, under providence, to the fidelity of husbands, wives, children, and servants, who braved the danger, and determined to obey the dictates of humanity." On the other hand, he noted that relatively "few of those who discharged their duty to their families" actually suffered for so doing.[15]

To counter the grim stories of cruelty and selfish neglect, Carey acknowledged "many illustrious instances, some in the middle, others in the lower spheres of life," of those who risked and sometimes sacrificed their lives to tend those in need, even strangers. "As a human being, I rejoice, that it has fallen to my lot, to be a witness and recorder of a magnanimity which would alone be sufficient to rescue the character of mortals from obloquy and reproach."[16] Nonetheless, however much Carey praised the virtues of admirable individuals, it is clear that their isolated actions were not in themselves sufficient to redeem the city from anarchy. It would require the collective efforts of public-spirited *citizens* to accomplish that.

At this lowest point, on 10 September, Mayor Clarkson, one of the few representatives of established authority who had not abandoned the city, "published an address to the citizens . . . inviting such benevolent people, as felt for the general distress, to lend their aid." Two days later a public meeting was held at the city hall. Only "a few" attended, but ten of those "offered themselves" to help the Guardians of the Poor, and a committee was appointed to inspect conditions at Bush Hill. This was found to be in "very bad order."[17] On the 14th, another public meeting determined to assume expanded social responsibilities. A committee of 26, "men mostly taken from the middle walks of life," was appointed, though because of death or desertion the bulk of the work was done by about 18. In Carey's words, this group's efforts "have been so highly favoured by providence, that they have been the instruments of averting the progress of destruction, eminently relieving the distressed, and restoring confidence to the terrified inhabitants of Philadelphia."[18] At this moment, Philadelphia was reborn as a community.

Carey's representation of this moment in which public order is restored, regenerated by the creation of a new social compact, refers back to previous constitutive moments in American civic mythology; among them the Mayflower Compact, the Declaration of Independence, and the Constitutional Convention. In this case, however, the creators of this emergency social contract had not been brought forward by divine or popular election. They were simply—in Carey's depiction, and it must be noted that he was one of the committee though he never mentions this fact—ordinary men, distinguished by their "benevolence" and their readiness to volunteer their services for the public good. Like Franklin's voluntary militia that had defended the city in 1748, they were common men responding to an uncommon emergency.[19] In Carey's telling, it was only after they voluntarily "offered themselves" that "providence" had "favoured" their efforts. Moreover, it is important to note that this was no purely Lockean, pragmatic social compact. The members of the committee recognized that more than mere convenience was at stake: the very survival of their city and perhaps their lives depended on reknitting the bonds of community.

This act of reconstitution of a new civic order was capped by a further remarkable development, "to which the most glowing pencil could hardly do justice." Two committee members who had seen the "deplorable" state of affairs at Bush Hill volunteered to take personal charge of the hospital. They were Stephen Girard, a French-born merchant and one of the wealthiest men in Philadelphia, who was to act as the "inside partner" of the hazardous enterprise, and Peter Helm, a native-born German-speaking cooper, who directed the outside tasks of transporting patients and supplies and burying the dead. Together, the merchant and the cooper brought order out of a nightmarish world that, according to Carey, through neglect, "riot and intemperance" among the nursing staff, had become "a great human slaughter house."[20] Soon the rooms were cleaned, patients grouped according to various stages of the disease, adequate supplies and nourishing food secured and disciplined care provided. In time, public confidence had so risen that people with illnesses other than the yellow fever were trying to get in.[21]

Meanwhile, the committee met each day from mid-September through November. In the abdication of all other authority, and by virtue of the authority granted it by the town meeting, this group of volunteers assumed "by tacit, but universal consent," all governmental functions.[22] They founded a home for the orphans of the fever and provided relief for those left penniless by the "stagnation of business." They appointed an extended "assistant committee of distribution" from the various districts of the city to identify those truly "deserving" of aid. As the disease gradually began to abate, the committee published notices prescribing measures for cleansing sites of illness and warning those in the country not to return prematurely.[23]

Day in and day out, committee members met at the city hall to deal with the needs of the moment. Carey described the "dreary" round of "fifteen, twenty, thirty applications daily, for coffins and carts to bury the dead, who had none to perform that last office for them—or as many applications for the removal of the sick to Bush hill." Despite these conditions, he noted that the committee "conducted their business with more harmony than is generally to be met with in public bodies of equal number."[24] Much later, he would recall the experience in his memoirs in even more positive terms, calling it one of the high points in his life.

> It is a curious fact, which I leave physiologists to account for, that some of the most tranquil and happy hours of my existence, were passed during the prevalence of this pestilence. And the feelings of my colleagues [on the committee] generally, were pretty much the same. I was for the first time for ten years, wholly free from the cares of business—had no money to borrow—no notes to pay—and my mind was fully occupied by the duties to which I had devoted myself. We generally breakfasted at home, at an early hour, and mustered immediately at the state house, where we remained till late in the evening. We had a sideboard plentifully provided . . . and we freely enjoyed the good things provided for us—became a band of brothers, attached to each other.[25]

How do we account for this astonishing admission, that this scene of death and despair was also experienced as a moment of tranquility and happiness? At one level, one can note the martial implications of his implied reference to Shakespeare's Henry V and his "band of brothers" at Agincourt. Towards the end of his pamphlet Carey employed a similar image when offering an "analogy" between Philadelphia and an army of recruits: both had been seized at the beginning by "an universal trepidation," but both in time became battle-hardened and behaved "with the most exemplary fortitude."[26] Over time, human beings can become inured to even the most horrifying of conditions.

More importantly, we can see here the intriguing story of an ambitious, struggling young entrepreneur who finds his greatest happiness in a moment when ordinary business pursuits can be put aside and his entire energies devoted to collective efforts toward a common good. At a mundane level, as Carey notes, in the cessation of business during the emergency he had "no notes to pay," and his correspondence at this time demonstrates that he had many at that very moment that he was hard pressed to pay. The disaster provided a rare moment of freedom from the personal striving and financial maneuvering that dominated his life as a publisher. But it is also clear that he derived a special satisfaction from working with others on a project that demanded all his attention, and in the service of what he could perceive as a public good. In fact, his description of the experience closely resembles what psychologist Mihaly Csikszentmihalyi has recently described as a state of "flow," in which a person becomes so absorbed in a complex task—whether physical, mental or social—that he or she loses all sense of time and of self-consciousness, yet experiences the greatest enjoyment.[27] Indeed, Carey seems to have been so affected by this experience that he sought to replicate it throughout the rest of his life, initiating and participating in a host of public committees and voluntary associations to improve and develop his adopted city, state, and nation. In his career as businessman and public-spirited citizen, Carey would serve as a model for nineteenth-century civic leaders seeking to balance republican ideals and expanding economic opportunities.

Carey's chronological retelling of events, followed by an encyclopedic array of anecdotes and numerical tables, can easily create the impression that he had indeed included "all the news fit to print" about the epidemic. Nonetheless, such an impression would be wrong, for Carey's narrative, like most, succeeds in telling one story about the epidemic by leaving out other possible stories. As the members of the African-American community learned to their chagrin when the first editions of Carey's *Short Account* appeared, he chose to all but ignore *their* heroic efforts during the emergency. According to Carey's ordering of events, public order had reached a nadir around 10 September when Mayor Clarkson gave his call to "benevolent" citizens to come forward. Yet several days earlier, on 5 September, the Free African Society had met to discuss Benjamin Rush's desperate plea that, because blacks were believed to be less vulnerable to the fever, they come forward to nurse the sick. The following day, African American leaders Absalom Jones and Richard Allen met with Clarkson and offered to coordinate the hiring of their people as nurses, gravediggers, and carters.[28] Carey ignored this excellent instance of voluntary community action, acknowledging only in the later section of anecdotes in his *Account* that blacks had served as nurses. Moreover, even while praising the great services of Jones, Allen, and William Gray, Carey devoted more space and much more vivid prose to invective for "some of the vilest of the black" who "extorted" unreasonably high wages and were accused of "plundering the houses of the sick." In a footnote, in the last edition, he admitted that many white nurses had also behaved badly.[29]

Why did Carey slight the contributions of African Americans? It may be, as has been argued, that as an Irish-born immigrant himself he was influenced by racism arising from the growing competition between Irish immigrants and free blacks for lesser skilled jobs.[30] But it may also be that he consciously or unconsciously perceived that doing full justice to the efforts of the Free African Society would undercut his dramatic narrative of community regeneration, focused as it was around the public meetings of 12 and 14 September. Whatever the case, it must be recognized that Carey's inspiring image of "public-spirited citizen" had no room for people of color, or for women. He touches upon the contribution of both blacks and women as *individuals*, but they appear in the narrative only as auxiliary figures (such as Mrs. Saville, the exemplary matron of Bush Hill, whom he recognizes by name only in a footnote in the last edition). He reserves his central roles as founding fathers of the new social compact for white, male middle-class citizens, who alone were eligible to participate fully in public life.

Allen and Jones were justifiably outraged at the way that Carey's *Account* had (literally) marginalized their contributions, for they had hoped through their sacrifices to gain recognition and acceptance as full members of the community. In response, they wrote their *own* version of events, *A Narrative of the Proceedings of the Black People, During the Late Awful Calamity in Philadelphia*, which attacked Carey's "partial representation" of their conduct.[31]

As this controversy demonstrates, many Philadelphians recognized that the story of how they had responded to this crisis was of more than passing interest. Viewed objectively, the yellow fever epidemic of 1793 was not the worst single epidemic in Philadelphia's or America's history, but because it occurred in the capital city at a formative time in the new nation's history, it carried symbolic weight far beyond the precise mortality figures.[32] In shaping his story as a dramatic narrative of community destruction and regeneration, Carey reflected and spoke to the volatile ideological and political moment of the 1790s. At the moment of the epidemic's inception, conflict had reached fever pitch between the newly established Federalist government and an emerging political coalition of those in "the middle walks of life": artisans, farmers, and fledgling manufacturers alike. Arriving from Ireland in 1785, Carey had at first championed the cause of strengthening the national government, but by 1793 he had begun to question the legitimacy of Hamiltonian programs that seemed to benefit only established elites.[33]

Like Benjamin Rush and Tench Coxe, other erstwhile supporters of the Constitution who became Jeffersonians in the 1790s, Carey adhered to ideas that can be categorized as *both* "liberal" and "republican."[34] He advocated a strong public sphere governed by virtuous, "public-spirited" citizens who placed the common good above partial private "interests"; but he also envisioned this world as animated by a dynamic entrepreneurial economy. In a departure from classical republicanism, Carey's public included not only gentlemen and planters, but "middling" tradesmen and artisans. In this charged political context, many of his contemporaries were acutely aware of the fact that, with the exception of Mayor Clarkson, the Federalist city government had abandoned the city during the crisis, and that middling citizens, generally excluded from leadership roles, had proved that they possessed at least as much virtue as their social betters.[35]

Carey's *Short Account* helped frame the way that Americans outside of Philadelphia thought about the epidemic's significance. For example, the first issue of the first newspaper in Cincinnati, Ohio, was dominated by a letter reprinted from the *Pittsburgh Gazette* about Philadelphia's epidemic—or, rather, Mathew Carey's account of it. The letter mirrored Carey's narrative, detailing the mortality, the desolation, and the hopeful denouement. "While physicians, magistrates, and people were flying from the devoted city, a generous band associated, to check the progress of the disease. . . ." The letter's author advocated that his readers emulate the committee's benevolence not only by contributing to the aid to the afflicted, but also by preferring Philadelphia manufactures and goods once trade resumed. He concluded, "let us avoid and have no dealings with those who meanly shrunk from the duties of humanity, and wrapping themselves up in the narrow bounds of their own wellfare, left their afflicted neighbors to misery, despair and death."[36]

Beyond its immediate significance, in telling a story of how benevolent citizens came forward to save their community, Carey contributed to the development of a broader paradigm of citizen voluntarism, in which the "people" themselves, not the state, band together in moments of public emergency and reknit "the bonds of society." Such extra-governmental activism contrasted with the customary modes of response to serious epidemics in Europe and colonial America. Even in severe cases such as the plagues in London in 1665 and Marseilles in 1720, public authorities not only remained in force but wielded extraordinary power to improve sanitation, to quarantine, to control commerce and even to array military force to contain residents within infected cities.[37] Carey's brief histories of these two plagues in an appendix implicitly contrasted Philadelphia's experiences with those of Europe.

This narrative of community destruction and regeneration has continued to influence the ways Americans have responded to (and have represented their response to) civic disasters. When disasters have struck, from floods in Cincinnati in 1832, to a hurricane in Galveston, Texas in 1900, to floods in the Mississippi River Valley in 1993, "citizens' committees" have come forward to restore public order and volunteers have gathered to fight back the waters and aid the victims.[38] In "The City That Saved Itself," sociolinguist Barbara Johnstone describes a remarkably similar narrative of citizen action told by residents and journalists in Fort Wayne, Indiana, about that city's response to a flood in 1982.[39] And in his 1995 State of the Union address, Bill Clinton praised the efforts of volunteers during recent flooding in California and urged, "Let's not wait for disasters to come together as a community."[40]

I would like to suggest that Carey's story of the creation of community through the public-spirited contributions of ordinary (albeit predominantly white, male) citizens also represents a foundation narrative in a civic mythology that has in the subsequent two centuries profoundly influenced the ways that Americans have thought about their relationship to civic life in general. Just as the experience of working on the committee launched Carey on a career of voluntary public service, his narrative promoted a vision of participatory, cooperative action for the public good that has long been an animating ideal in American life. Because it has been such a powerful narrative, it is all the more regrettable that Carey failed to include all of those who contributed to his city's regeneration. It is therefore all the more important to recognize today the ways in which the construction of Carey's narrative marginalized some members of the community in order to bring others to center stage.

NOTES

1. John H. Powell, *Bring Out Your Dead: The Great Plague of Yellow Fever in Philadelphia in 1793* (Philadelphia: University of Pennsylvania Press, 1949), pp. 42–43. This full-length account relies heavily on Carey's dramatic narrative.

2. Eve Kornfeld argues that the various reactions to the epidemic revealed attitudes toward the new national culture, "Crisis in the Capital: The Cultural Significance of Philadelphia's Great Yellow Fever Epidemic," *Pennsylvania History* 51 (1984): 189–205. On New England interpretations of dramatic events as providential, see David D. Hall, *Worlds of Wonder, Days of Judgment: Popular Religious Belief in Early New England* (New York: Alfred A. Knopf, 1989); and David Paul Nord, "Teleology and News: The Religious Roots of American Journalism, 1630–1730," *Journal of American History* 77 (1990): 9–38.

3. Nord discusses the relationship between the doctrine of divine providence and the development of "a particular methodology for identifying, gathering, reporting, and publishing news stories" in "Teleology and News," p. 38.

4. He had already published a much briefer account, *A Desultory Account of the Yellow Fever, Prevalent in Philadelphia, and of the Present State of the City* (Philadelphia: Mathew Carey, 1793) on 16 October.

5. Mathew Carey to James Carey, 6 April 1794, Mathew Carey Letterbooks, B-45, Lea and Febiger Collection, Historical Society of Pennsylvania.

6. Carey's activities and accomplishments were so diverse that there has been no single comprehensive treatment of his life. A useful general overview is provided by James N. Green in *Mathew Carey: Publisher and Patriot* (Philadelphia: The Library Company of Philadelphia, 1985). Other works include Edward C. Carter II, "The Political Activities of Mathew Carey, Nationalist, 1760–1814" (Ph.D. diss., Bryn Mawr College, 1962), and "Mathew Carey and 'The Olive Branch,' 1814–1818," *Pennsylvania Magazine of History and Biography* 89 (1965): 399–415; Earl L. Bradsher, *Mathew Carey, Editor, Author and Publisher: A Study in American Literary Development* (New York: Columbia University Press, 1912); and Kenneth W. Rowe, *Mathew Carey: A Study in American Economic Development* (Baltimore: Johns Hopkins University Press, 1933).

7. Mathew Carey, *A Short Account of the Malignant Fever, Lately Prevalent in Philadelphia*, 4th ed., improved (1794; reprint, New York: Arno Press, 1970), p. 10. All subsequent references are to this edition.

8. Ibid., p. 11. Other accounts of the epidemic focused more exclusively on its providential cause, including Justus Henry Christian Helmuth, *Short Account of the Yellow Fever in Philadelphia, for the Reflecting Christian* (Philadelphia: Printed by Jones, Hoff, and Derrick, 1794), and Samuel Stearns, *An Account of the Terrible Effects of the Pestilential Infection in the City of Philadelphia* (Providence: Printed for William Child, 1793).

9. Carey, *Short Account*, pp. 16, 17.

10. Ibid., pp. 18–19, 30.

11. Ibid., p. 22. For a detailed examination of the role of Brown's *Federal Gazette* in the 1793 epidemic, see David Paul Nord's essay in this volume.

12. Carey, *Short Account*, p. 22.

13. Ibid., p. 23.

14. Mathew Carey, *Autobiography* (New York: E.L. Schwaab, 1942), p. 26.

15. Carey, *Short Account*, pp. 72–73.

16. Ibid., pp. 27–28.

17. Ibid., pp. 28–29.

18. Ibid., p. 30.

19. Sally F. Griffith, " 'Order, Discipline, and a few Cannon': Benjamin Franklin, The Association, and the Rhetoric and Practice of Boosterism," *Pennsylvania Magazine of History and Biography* 116 (1992): 131–155.

20. Carey, *Short Account*, p. 32.

21. Ibid., p. 34.

22. Ibid., p. 30.

23. Ibid., pp. 35–39.

24. Ibid., pp. 43, 30.

25. Carey, *Autobiography*, 27.

26. Carey, *Short Account*, 92.

27. Mihaly Csikszentmihalyi, *Flow: The Psychology of Optimal Experience* (New York: Harper and Row, 1990).

28. For the contributions of Philadelphia's African-Americans in the epidemic, see Gary Nash, *Forging Freedom: The Formation of Philadelphia's Black Community, 1720–1840* (Cambridge, Mass.: Harvard University Press, 1988), pp. 122–125; and Phillip Lapsansky's essay in this volume.

29. Carey, *Short Account*, p. 63.

30. This is Nash's argument; see *Forging Freedom*, p. 125.

31. Absalom Jones and Richard Allen, *A Narrative of the Proceedings of the Black People, During the Late Awful Calamity in Philadelphia, in the Year 1793: and a Refutation of Some Censures, Thrown Upon Them in Some Late Publications* (1794; reprint, Philadelphia: Independence National Historical Park, 1993).

32. Paul Slack has pointed out that the reaction to epidemics often bears no logical relation to the morbidity or mortality, but is affected by the particular characteristics of the disease and broader cultural factors, in his introduction to Paul Slack and Terence Ranger, eds., *Epidemics and Ideas: Essays on the Historical Perception of Pestilence* (Cambridge: Cambridge University Press, 1992).

33. John R. Nelson, Jr., *Liberty and Property: Political Economy and Policymaking in the New Nation, 1789–1812* (Baltimore: Johns Hopkins University Press, 1987), p. xiv

and passim; Cathy D. Matson and Peter S. Onuf, *A Union of Interests: Political and Economic Thought in Revolutionary America* (Lawrence: University Press of Kansas, 1990); John E. Crowley, *The Privileges of Independence: Neomercantilism and the American Revolution* (Baltimore: Johns Hopkins University Press, 1993), pp. 146–154. Foreign relations also played a part in Carey's shift: he had been among a group of thirty prominent Republicans who welcomed Citizen Genêt in May, 1793. Roland M. Baumann, "The Democratic-Republicans of Philadelphia: The Origins, 1776–1797" (Ph.D. diss., Pennsylvania State University, 1970), p. 427. On the connection between political ideology and the response to the 1793 epidemic, see Martin Pernick's 1972 essay reprinted in this volume.

34. Recently the long debate over whether liberalism *or* republicanism shaped the nation's founding has begun to be recast in a recognition that both traditions were part of the discursive repertoire of colonial and early-national political actors. See discussions in Matson and Onuf, *Union of Interests*, pp. 2, 11–12.

35. Ronald Schultz emphasizes the class dimension of the 1793 epidemic, and the artisanal character of the Committee, in *Republic of Labor: Philadelphia Artisans and the Politics of Class, 1720–1830* (New York: Oxford University Press, 1993), pp. 134–137, 264n.

36. *Centinel of the North-Western Territory*, 28 December 1793.

37. Paul Slack, "Responses to Plague in Early Modern Europe: The Implications of Public Health" in *In Time of Plague: The History and Social Consequences of Lethal Epidemic Disease* (New York: New York University Press, 1991), pp. 111–131. Little has been written on government responses to epidemics in colonial America, but descriptions of particular episodes suggest that colonial governments made similar efforts to prevent the spread of infectious diseases. In New England and the Middle Colonies, fast days were also decreed in an attempt to forestall divine wrath. See Geoffrey Marks and William K. Beatty, *Epidemics* (New York: Charles Scribner's Sons, 1976), pp. 149–156; John Duffy, *Epidemics in Colonial America* (Baton Rouge: Louisiana State University Press, 1953); and Hall, *Worlds of Wonder*, pp. 168–172.

38. Examples of histories that feature such heroic interpretations are: Charles Frederic Goss, *Cincinnati: The Queen City, 1788–1912* (Chicago and Cincinnati: S. J. Clarke Publishing Company, 1912), pp. 586–587; Herbert Molloy Mason, Jr., *Death from the Sea: Our Greatest Natural Disaster, the Galveston Hurricane of 1900* (New York: Dial Press, 1972), pp. 182–201; and David G. McComb, *Galveston: A History* (Austin: University of Texas Press, 1986), pp. 127–130. In Galveston, the increased class and racial conflicts of the late nineteenth century were also reflected in preoccupations with looting by blacks and immigrants.

39. Barbara Johnstone, *Stories, Community and Place* (Bloomington: Indiana University Press, 1990), chapter 6.

40. Press Release, Office of the Press Secretary, "Remarks by the President in the State of the Union Address, January 24, 1995."

"Abigail, a Negress": The Role and the Legacy of African Americans in the Yellow Fever Epidemic

PHILLIP LAPSANSKY

MONG the many texts emanating from the yellow fever epidemic of 1793 is an account of the efforts of Philadelphia African Americans during these troubled months, written by the black clergymen and community leaders Richard Allen and Absalom Jones. *A Narrative of the Proceedings of the Black People, During the Late Awful Calamity in Philadelphia, in the Year 1793: And a Refutation of Some Censures, Thrown upon Them in Some Late Publications* was published in Philadelphia in January of 1794, a scant two months after the fever had run its course. The *Narrative* is a major and important work in African American literature. It is the first account of a free black community in action, a first-hand account of the work of black Philadelphians among the sick and dying. It is also the first African American polemic in which black leaders sought to articulate black community anger and directly confront an accuser. The *Narrative* was written, seemingly, in reply to part of a paragraph in Mathew Carey's best-seller, *A Short Account of the Malignant Fever Lately Prevalent in Philadelphia.*[1] This essay revisits the *Narrative* as an artifact of the struggles of the first generation of free blacks in Philadelphia, and notes the influence and impact of the text, and its authors and subjects, on later generations of African Americans. "The elders of the African church met, and offered their services to the mayor, to procure nurses for the sick, and to assist in burying the dead," Carey wrote.

> Their offers were accepted; and Absalom Jones and Richard Allen undertook the former department . . . and William Gray, the latter. The great demand for nurses afforded an opportunity for imposition, which was eagerly seized by some of the vilest of the blacks. They extorted two, three, four, even five dollars a night for attendance, which would have been well paid by a single dollar. Some of them were even detected in plundering the houses of the sick. But it is wrong to cast a censure on the

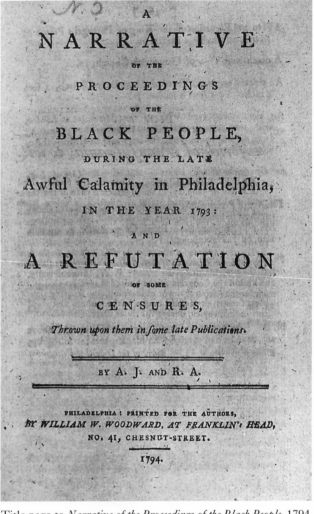

A

NARRATIVE

OF THE

PROCEEDINGS

OF THE

BLACK PEOPLE,

DURING THE LATE

Awful Calamity in Philadelphia,

IN THE YEAR 1793:

AND

A REFUTATION

OF SOME

CENSURES,

Thrown upon them in some late Publications.

BY A. J. AND R. A.

PHILADELPHIA : PRINTED FOR THE AUTHORS,
BY *WILLIAM W. WOODWARD, AT FRANKLIN's HEAD,*
NO. 41, CHESNUT-STREET.

1794.

Title page to *Narrative of the Proceedings of the Black People*, 1794.
Courtesy of the Library Company of Philadelphia.

whole for this sort of conduct, as many people have done. The services of Jones, Allen, and Gray, and others of their colour, have been very great, and demand public gratitude.[2]

Mathew Carey no doubt thought he had written a careful and balanced account, acknowledging the bad but praising the good, and admonishing his readers against casting "a censure on the whole." To the black leaders Richard Allen and Absalom Jones it was an example of the slavery-inspired every-day racism that dismissed black effort and opportunity. The charges of extortion and pilferage offended them, as did Carey's further remarks that dismissed the effects of the fever upon blacks, and sketched them as the grim heralds of death, terror, panic, and social disintegration, "The corpses of the most respectable citizens," Carey wrote, "were carried to the grave, on the shafts of a chair, the horse driven by a negro, unattended by a friend or relation, and without any sort of ceremony." He went on: "Many men of affluent fortunes have been abandoned to the care of a negro, after their wives, children, friends, clerks, and servant, had fled away, and left them to their fate."[3]

Especially painful was Carey's dismissive waffling on the supposed immunity of blacks to the fever. "They did not escape the disorder," Carey wrote, "however, the number of them that were seized with it, was not great; and, as I am informed by an eminent doctor, 'it yielded to the power of medicine in them more easily than in the whites.' " However, this mistaken notion of black immunity "had a very salutary effect," wrote Carey, "for at an early period of the disorder, hardly any white nurses could be procured; and had the negroes been equally terrified, the sufferings of the sick, great as they actually were, would have been exceedingly aggravated."[4]

To Jones, Allen, and their black constituents, it was intolerable that this should be the summary of their relief efforts during the epidemic. What had they, in fact, done?

In early September 1793 the city officials, citizens, and physicians who mobilized to confront the epidemic appealed to Jones, Allen, and other leaders of Philadelphia's free black community to aid in the relief effort. Physicians and most others believed blacks were immune to the disease and thus obliged to come to the aid of the afflicted. We do not know how widespread this idea was among blacks, particularly those born and raised in or near Pennsylvania, such as Allen, Jones, and many of their colleagues.

Heeding their Christian commitment to mutual aid, the two black leaders, along with William Gray, Cyrus Bustill, and others mobilized the foot soldiers in the war against the epidemic from Philadelphia's black population. These humblest of Philadelphians, many recently slaves, helped administer what was effectively the government of the city. As John Powell wrote of them, they "assumed the most onerous, the most disgusting burdens of demoralized whites."[5] They recruited nurses to visit homes and work at the Bush Hill hospital, mobilized carters to transport patients and remove the dead, enlisted laborers to dig the graves, and—for good or ill—administered Benjamin Rush's bleeding and purging treatment to hundreds of sufferers. They patrolled the streets, checked abandoned properties, and tried to maintain a semblance of social order.

The only agreed-upon remedy was flight, but most blacks stayed. Some

750 blacks lived in the areas most affected by the fever. About 40 percent of the whites fled this area, but only about 14 percent of the blacks.[6] But how mobile, how free, were these blacks? It is likely many were bound to a master or employer, one of the dwindling number of slaves, or a former slave indentured for a term of years. But many slaves, Philadelphians included, had always managed to flee, and what better reason than doctor's orders? Also, the disease, social disintegration and collapse of authority Carey details probably "freed" many blacks, who found themselves bound to dead, dying, or absent masters. Some, like Allen and Jones, were property owners and perhaps reluctant to leave, though property-owning whites certainly were not.[7]

Perhaps in facetious tribute, the *Federal Gazette* ran a waggish dialogue between two Jersey farmers in which George tells William of his recent trip to the city to sell his goods at inflated prices. "The best news, and that from the Negroes, for they only come to Market now! They told me that 14,200 have already died—29,000 have gone out of town—so that only 1,425 people remain." William replies, "Your account is indeed a black one."[8]

The official praise of Mayor Clarkson and others in the wake of the epidemic must have been gratifying to blacks. But Carey's remarks were stinging and dangerous, defaming the struggling black community that had rallied itself to serve the city. Jones' and Allen's *Narrative* was their defense, and their attack.

Jones and Allen acknowledged that Carey had singled them out and praised their efforts, but they found his work essentially insulting to Philadelphia blacks and dismissive of the efforts of the mass of anonymous black workers Jones and Allen represented. "By naming us he leaves these others in the hazardous state of being classed with those who are called the vilest," they wrote. The stakes for blacks were high. "We have many unprovoked enemies who begrudge us the liberty we enjoy and are glad to hear of any complaints against our colour."[9]

In a sort of parallel text, Jones and Allen complemented Carey's many instances of cruelty and opportunism with accounts of individual black heroism and sacrifice. And, in mentioning only a few individuals, they underscored the important role of ordinary, unnamed black citizens. They told the story of life on the stricken streets, and of blacks who served for little or no pay, encountering the hostility and the fear of the whites they attempted to help. They wrote of the sheer hard work of it all. "Thus were many of the nurses circumstanced," they wrote, "alone, until the patient died, then called away to another scene of distress, and thus have been for a week or ten days left to do the best they could without sufficient rest, many of them having some of their dearest connexions sick at the time and suffering for want while their husband, wife, father, mother have been engaged in the service of the white people."[10]

How many blacks were involved in the relief effort? There are no hard numbers. Jones and Allen at this time were in direct contact with about 300 individual blacks, and they note that the number of black nurses was "twenty times" that of whites.[11] Whatever their number, their role was critical and central. When blacks began regularly to succumb to the fever, Benjamin Rush for one was in despair. "Negroes are everywhere submitting to the disorder," he wrote. "If it should spread among them, then will the measure of our suffering be full."[12]

Carey's charges of extortion and theft were most damaging, and Jones and Allen noted it was whites who drove up the prices, outbidding each other for the services of black nurses—the same simple forces of supply and demand that Carey noted had driven Philadelphia rents steadily upward, though he never described landlords as "the vilest." Rush, in fact, joked about this competition for black services with one of the nurses: "Hah! Mama!" he exclaimed, "We black folks have come into demand at last." Moreover, they were angered that Carey's account seemed to emphasize black theft and pilferage, while ignoring the criminal behavior of many whites. "It is that they only are pointed out, and made mention of, we esteem partial and injurious."[13]

Jones and Allen denounced Carey's charges and threw them back at him. "Had Mr. Carey been solicited to such an undertaking," they asked, "what would he have demanded? We believe he has made more money by the sale of his scraps [i.e., his pamphlet] than a dozen of the greatest extortioners among the black nurses." They included in their narrative an accounting of the money and property that came into their hands, and noted that blacks spent 177 pounds of their own money in the effort and expected no recompense.[14]

Some two hundred years later, novelist John Edgar Wideman, in a short story, wrote of the situation of the Philadelphia blacks of 1793 in the fictionalized first person voice of a participant.

> Why did I not fly? Why was I not dancing in the streets, celebrating God's judgment on this wicked city? Fever made me freer than I'd ever been. Municipal government had collapsed. Anarchy ruled. As long as fever did not strike me I could come and go anywhere I pleased. Fortunes could be made in the streets. I could sell myself to the highest bidder, as nurse or undertaker, as surgeon trained by the famous Dr. Rush to apply his lifesaving cure. . . . To be spared the fever was a chance for anyone, black or white, to be a king.[15]

As Wideman suggests, and as Carey could infer from his own description of the collapse of civil authority, the only force keeping blacks in town and in service was their own self-discipline and commitment.

Particularly painful was Carey's dismissive remarks on the impact of the fever upon blacks, and Jones and Allen replied with angry passion. "When the people of colour had the sickness and died, we were imposed upon and told it

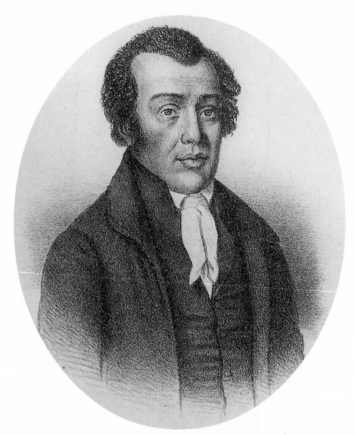

Portrait of the Reverend Richard Allen, n.d. Courtesy of the Library Company of Philadelphia.

was not with the prevailing sickness, until it became too notorious to be denied, then we were told some few died but not many. Thus were our services extorted at the peril of our lives, yet you accuse us of extorting a little money from you."[16] We wonder if Allen wrote this particular passage. He contracted yellow fever in late October and recovered after three weeks in Bush Hill, under the care of the black attendants he himself helped recruit.[17]

It is likely a few blacks, seamen and laborers in the streets and alleys of the river front, were among the earliest fever victims. As the fever progressed through September and October, blacks probably suffered from it as much as the whites. Some blacks, as some whites, were immune by prior exposure to the fever—those dwindling number of Africans or those from parts of the

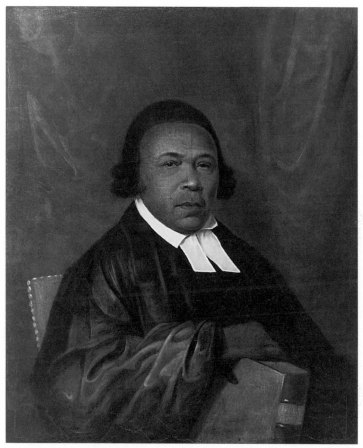

Absalom Jones, 1810, by Raphaelle Peale. Courtesy of the Delaware Art Museum, gift of the Absalom Jones School.

West Indies where yellow fever was prevalent. But as Philadelphia blacks knew, their community was increasingly an African American community, and the native born, or those from nearby states, were no more immune to yellow fever than the whites. Also, though the concept of "seasoning" or acclimation was probably known to many blacks, we do not know how many really believed in their immunity, nor what credit they gave white authorities who declared it so. According to one estimate, the fever struck 11 percent of the blacks and 14 percent of the whites, a statistically significant difference, but the meaning of it was probably lost in life on the suffering streets.

Black fever fatalities are estimated at 198. Recorded black burials for 1793 totaled 305, up from 67 for the previous year.[18] Jones and Allen name only two black victims, nurses Sampson and Caesar Cranchall. Another dozen or so are listed in the Bush Hill records.[19] And, by accident of alphabetical order, at the head of a list of the dead appended to the fourth edition of Carey's account is "Abigail, a Negress."[20] Who was she? I confess I do not know. I have yet to find her in any of the other surviving records.[21] Possibly she was one of the 50 percent of Philadelphia blacks who were live-in workers. Maybe she was one of the 200 or so who were still slaves in the city. Perhaps she was a fugitive, or recently freed in a neighboring slave state, or brought from St. Domingue with her fleeing master—one of many such migrants who swelled Philadelphia's black population from just under 3,000 in 1790 to around 3,300 in 1793 and over 6,000 in 1800. We meet Abigail only in Carey's list of the dead, where she is joined by "Barbe, a black woman," "Dick, a negro," "Flora, a black girl," "Juliana, a Mulatto," "Timothy, a black man"—the half-names and labels by which so many Philadelphia blacks were known. "We have suffered equally with the whites," Jones and Allen wrote of their mostly anonymous dead. "Our distress has been very great, but much unknown to the white people. Few have been the whites who paid attention to us."[22]

But the lesson of Abigail's mortality was not lost on whites. An account of the 1797 yellow fever epidemic notes: "The College of Physicians recommended, in preference, as nurses to the sick, Negroes who were natives of Africa. This produced an inconvenience; for, the blacks of this country became alarmed, and generally refused to attend; while the scarcity of Africans, made people bid high for them, and raised, to exorbitance, the price of their attendance." But in spite of the ill-will, black Philadelphian Richard Allen was again on the streets during the 1797 epidemic. Did he know his bout with the fever in 1793 made him immune in 1797? If not, then he served in the face of a threat that, from intimate and personal experience, he felt he had every reason to fear.[23]

Jones and Allen identified slavery as the source of racist opinion and denigration and wrote the sharpest attack on the cruel hypocrisy of slaveholder ideology yet published by African Americans. It is foolish, they argued, "that a superior good conduct is looked for, from our race, by those who stigmatize us as men, whose baseness is incurable, and may therefore be held in a state of servitude, yet you try what you can to prevent our rising from the state of barbarism you represent us to be in. But we can tell you," they continued, "that a black man, although reduced to the most abject state human nature is capable of, short of real madness, can think, reflect, and feel injuries, although it may not be with the same degree of resentment and revenge that you who have been and are our great oppressors would manifest if reduced to the pitiable condition of a slave."[24]

In four paragraphs addressed "To the People of Colour," Jones and Allen wrote of the hard truths that confronted blacks, mostly despised and hopelessly outnumbered. Themselves former slaves, Jones and Allen extended their sympathy to those still in bondage and urged Christian love and forbearance, for "no master can deprive you of it." They reiterated the persistent admonition to good behavior in a hostile climate where any individual shortcoming of any particular black would be ascribed to the race as a whole. "If we are lazy and idle, the enemies of freedom plead it as a cause why we ought not to be free. By such conduct we strengthen the bands of oppression. Will even our friends, will God pardon us, for the part we act in making strong the hands of the enemies of our colour."[25]

The two black leaders concluded their narrative with a paragraph of praise and gratitude for the work of the antislavery whites. "You blow the trumpet against the mighty evil, you make the tyrants tremble; you strive to raise the slave, to the dignity of a man; you take our children by the hand, to lead them in the path of virtue, by your care of their education; you are not ashamed to call the most abject of our race, brethren, children of one father, who made of one blood all the nations of the earth."[26]

Carey was angered and insulted by the *Narrative*. He was a dedicated republican, with seemingly impeccable eighteenth-century antislavery credentials. His magazine, *The American Museum*, regularly featured antislavery and anti-slave-trade articles and occasional writings by blacks such as Phillis Wheatley and Prince Hall. And in his yellow fever pamphlet he had in fact praised Allen, Jones, and Gray by name. "I would fain ask the reader," Carey wrote in his defense, "is this the language of an enemy? Does this deserve railing or reproach? Is it honorable for Jones and Allen to repay evil for good?"[27]

Carey had missed the point. If the selfless efforts of this unnamed mass of most humble Philadelphians could be minimized and dismissed, what hope was there for the wider acceptance of blacks as freemen and citizens? Perhaps some of the blacks, at the height of the epidemic, had read the effusive essay in the *Federal Gazette*, probably a space filler, on "that godlike afection" benevolence: "To visit the abodes of wretchedness, to enter into the feelings of the unfortunate, to sympathize with their sorrows, and to relieve their distresses, are actions truly elevating and ennobling. . . . The honor due to actions of benevolence is more desireable, as it is inaccessible to the malignant shafts of envy."[28] And, perhaps, they thought these sentiments applied to them.

For the black leaders, Carey's pamphlet was one more insult they had faced in their efforts of the last several years to forge a viable community out of the partially free, randomly assembled black population, a struggle in which they confronted the racism and denigration that Carey seemed to articulate as common truth and conventional wisdom.

For years prior to 1793 Philadelphia free blacks had worked to establish an organizational community life for themselves. In 1787, Jones, Allen, and several other blacks founded the Free African Society, which served first as a beneficial society but quickly grew into a religious, mission-like organization promoting morality and discipline among blacks. Along with providing financial aid for the sick and disabled, the group also encouraged marriages, family formation, and organized religious life. As W.E.B. Du Bois wrote of this movement a century later, "it was the first wavering step of a people toward organized social life."[29] From the Free African Society came not only the cadre that worked so diligently during the 1793 epidemic, but also the first independent black churches, both the focus and the generators of black community organization. The Free Africans divided denominationally. Richard Allen and those blacks inclined with him towards Methodism established Bethel Church in an abandoned blacksmith's shack. Absalom Jones and his followers organized the African Episcopal Church of St. Thomas, their newly built brick structure on 5th Street finally completed in 1794.[30]

The free black community that began to pull itself together in a self-organized fashion in the late 1780s clearly took roots in fertile soil. Though slavery flourished in early Philadelphia, so did antislavery. From the early antislavery protest of the Germantown Mennonites in 1688, through the antislavery writings of Ralph Sandiford in the 1720s, Benjamin Lay in the 1730s, John Woolman and Anthony Benezet in the 1750s and 1760s, and John Wesley and Benjamin Rush in the 1770s, Philadelphia presses produced a steady stream of antislavery literature in the pre-Revolutionary period.[31]

Some Philadelphia slaves, such as Absalom Jones, no doubt learned to read from sympathetic masters and ministers; these individual attempts were supplemented by sporadic organized efforts. In 1723, the Quaker reformer Samuel Keimer established a school "to teach his poor Brethren the Male Negroes to read the Holy Scriptures."[32] The British philanthropists of the Bray Associates, linking literacy to salvation, established a school for blacks in 1758. And most notable was the career of Quaker educator Anthony Benezet, who began tutoring blacks around 1750 and continued to his death in 1784.[33]

Antislavery concern and protest had by the mid-1760s ended the direct African slave trade to Philadelphia ports. And in 1775, antislavery Philadelphians, largely Quakers, organized the nation's first antislavery society, the Pennsylvania Society for Promoting the Abolition of Slavery (PAS). After the American Revolution, the Society was reconstituted as a larger and more diverse group, including such notables as Benjamin Rush, a member since 1784; Benjamin Franklin, the Society's President in his last years; and, by 1797, Mathew Carey. Seemingly widespread antislavery sentiment led to the passage of Pennsylvania's gradual emancipation act in 1780, and antislavery forces continued to struggle against slavery and the slave trade in the new nation. They celebrated examples of black talent such as poet Phillis Wheatley, physician James Durham, mathematician Thomas Fuller, and Benjamin Banneker, whose almanacs were issuing from the presses of sympathetic

Philadelphia printers. They supported schools for blacks, and in 1793 blacks secured the appointment of one of their own, Helena Harris, as a teacher.[34] They provided legal aid, and helped secure indentures to provide employment. And their association with like-minded groups in other states portended a successful national antislavery effort. Indeed they were valuable allies, and were regarded by black leaders as the most hopeful sign of the possibilities of interracial justice.[35]

But the white antislavery movement was not enough. More important were the black community-building organizations that provided social and psychological nurture and support in a hostile racial environment, and articulated the blacks' point of view on important issues affecting them. These, blacks learned, only they could build. And, they learned, their efforts to do and to speak for themselves angered paternalistic whites who saw blacks as fit objects for comforting benevolence but not for self-confident independence. Philadelphia blacks came to appreciate the limits and fatuity of gradualist antislavery sentiment. They knew that Pennsylvania's much-heralded emancipation act was basically a slaveholders' measure which extended servitude for many years. While changing economic circumstances made slavery less profitable and led many to free their slaves, most freed blacks worked themselves free through years of labor. Both Jones and Allen were such self-freed slaves, and Jones served well into middle age to buy himself and his wife. In the quibbles and caveats of the time, they saw Pennsylvania slaveholders cling tenaciously to their black property, or sell them to the South. Even allies like Benjamin Rush kept a slave as a personal servant. Blacks knew that through their extended servitude they bore the costs and burdens of emancipation.[36]

Also, among sympathetic whites, antislavery was increasingly becoming coupled with ideas of black removal.[37] In 1787, the British established the West African outpost of Sierra Leone to which they shipped blacks from Great Britain and black refugees in their charge from the American revolutionary wars. Americans quickly followed with schemes for African resettlement and other plans for mass black relocation in the American southwest or some other distant corner of the continent. Steadily, ideas of some sort of resettlement elsewhere gained popularity among many abolitionists and chipped away at the possibilities of black citizenship. While ideas of African resettlement enjoyed some popularity in other northern black communities, the Free Africans were more hopeful of their possibilities as African Americans and black Philadelphians. Further, as underscored in the *Narrative*, free black Philadelphians saw their destiny linked to the slaves' and would not consider abandoning them. The social progress of the Free Africans would serve as an inspiration to those in bondage and prove to the larger society the possibilities of black freedom.[38]

To ideas and schemes for the physical removal of blacks were attached notions of their genetic removal as well. Enlightened eighteenth-century opinion regarded race, as manifest in skin color, a matter of environment that did, and could again, change. The conventional wisdom of the times is detailed in Thomas Dobson's *Encyclopaedia*: "If whites be considered as the stock from whence all others have sprung, it is easy to conceive how they have degenerated into negroes." And, in reverse: "A much greater length of time is undoubtably necessary before negroes, when transplanted into our temperate countries, can entirely lose their black colour. By crossing the breed with whites, every taint of the negro colour may be expelled, we believe, from the fifth generation." Thus the only important question was whether the characteristics of blacks, defined as "idleness, treachery, revenge, cruelty, impudence, stealing, lying, profanity, debauchery, nastiness and intemperance," were innate qualities or the consequences of such brutalizing social environments as African "barbarism" and American slavery.[39]

Other events in the years prior to the epidemic further convinced Philadelphia blacks of their need to focus attention on creating independent community-building organizations through which to act and, particularly, speak for themselves. In 1790, blacks saw the antislavery optimism of the revolutionary age falter in the defeat of abolition legislation in Congress, compromised away by legislators who regarded themselves as good antislavery men. In September of 1792, in what might have been a petulant response to black organization, black worshippers at St. George Methodist Church were rudely informed of new rules requiring their segregation. As Absalom Jones knelt in prayer at the altar, whites attempted to drag him away, telling him he could not worship there. "Wait until prayer is over, and I will get up and trouble you no more," Jones replied, and led a walkout of several black members.[40]

Blacks were bitterly disappointed in 1793 with the passage of the Fugitive Slave Act. Some were themselves fugitives, hopefully settled beyond the reach of their former masters. Many had family members still in slavery, and the prospect of escape was also a prospect for family reunification. The new law also served as a cover to the growing practice of kidnapping free blacks to sell into slavery, a practice that soon became something of a cottage industry among unscrupulous whites. In the following years, as a community spokesman, Absalom Jones repeatedly denounced the injustice of the law in petitions and memorials to Congress.[41]

As their organizing efforts advanced, blacks met mostly with white anger and resentment and were accused of arrogance, pride and ingratitude. In the summer of 1793, as blacks attempted to raise $3,000 to build what became St. Thomas Church, they found white philanthropy tight-fisted, but witnessed a sudden outpouring of charity for the slaveholding refugees from Cape François, fleeing the slave rebellion in St. Domingue. It must have been galling to see these same whites, hostile to the support of a local church, give over

$12,000 in just a few days for the relief of slaveholders. And what to blacks were these shiploads of refugees but more slave ships, for many of the refugees brought their personal slaves.

The *Narrative* is the voice of years of experience with these various forces and events shaping their lives. And from these experiences, brought into sharp focus by the dismissive disregard of their efforts in the yellow fever crisis, came an intensified commitment to build the black organizations that helped integrate their rapidly growing population into a community. With the completion of St. Thomas in 1794, about 400 black Philadelphians, drawn from some 350 black families, were organized into the two new churches, and they struggled for years against white opinion and the efforts of church authorities to keep these fledgling organizations under their control. St. Thomas won its autonomy in a compromise with Episcopal authorities that barred the congregation from participating in the Church's governing councils. Allen's Methodist church faced a tougher, longer fight, wrangling for years with Methodist authorities who tried to seize control of their ministry and membership. Finally, in 1816, Allen, joined by other recently formed black congregations, turned away from the Methodist establishment and organized a separate black denomination, the African Methodist Episcopal Church, the first truly national African American organization. The two churches spawned a variety of organizations to support the sick, to promote education through black schools and literary societies, and to provide community definition through fraternal organizations and social and mission groups.[42] St. Thomas and Bethel Church continue today as active, vital, and venerable ministries.

The men and women of 1793 became the leaders of a growing and diverse black population, many of whom prospered as artisans, craftsmen, and businessmen, laying the basis of an economically secure middle class able to further promote and fund black community organizations and to articulate their views on important issues. Absalom Jones was finally officially ordained in 1804, becoming the first African American priest. His ministry is best known for actively promoting black education and, with Richard Allen and James Forten, he was one of the principal spokesmen of the African American community. Jones headed St. Thomas Church until his death in 1818. Richard Allen was always a leading figure in the Philadelphia community and, after 1816 and his ordination as first Bishop of the African Methodist Episcopal Church, he became the first African American leader of national stature. James Forten was part of the relief effort of 1793, a young man working in the riverfront sail loft he would soon own. He became one of the wealthiest Philadelphians, a long-time black community leader and spokesman until his death in 1842, a founder of the American Anti-Slavery Society, and the progenitor of several generations of African American intellectuals, writers, educators, and political leaders. And Frank Johnson, an infant in 1793, survived to become the first nationally renowned African American musician.[43]

As antiblack sentiment mounted in Philadelphia in the nineteenth century, as proscription and violence against blacks became commonplace, this black middle class was denounced, derided, dismissed, cartooned, and lampooned, but through their organized efforts they developed a black community known nationally among African Americans for its high level of education and culture. And the principles of this first generation of free black leaders, as articulated in the *Narrative*—their first public presentation—resonate through the words and deeds of nineteenth-century black Philadelphia.

Old antislavery allies were remembered and commemorated. When Benjamin Rush died in 1813, blacks buried him with rhetorical style and established in his honor the Rush Educational Society. A generation later, in 1836, young black intellectuals also remembered him in founding the Rush Library and Debating Society.[44] The slave revolution in St. Domingue that brought so many refugees, and probably the yellow fever, reverberated through black Philadelphia. They took interest and pride in the creation of Haiti as the first nation founded by self-liberated black slaves—for whom yellow fever was an ally that helped defeat the French troops sent against them. In 1818, Philadelphia blacks welcomed Haitian King Christophe's African American emissary Prince Saunders, and they listened with interest to his appeal for skilled and educated blacks to settle in Haiti. In the mid-1820s, Allen, Forten, and others promoted a program of Haitian emigration and some 200 Philadelphia blacks resettled in the new black nation.[45]

Though the Free Africans did not support the early schemes for returning blacks to Africa, interest in black-controlled emigration, resettlement beyond the reach of American slavery and racism, ebbed and flowed through nineteenth-century Philadelphia. Paul Cuffe, the African American ship captain who promoted settlement and trade to Sierra Leone, was a friend of many Philadelphia black leaders who were supportive of his efforts. But white-controlled colonization, which denied or decried black citizenship, was roundly rejected. In 1817, the American Colonization Society characterized free blacks as a degenerate and unassimilable group and urged, as an act of Christian charity, a national program for their removal to an African colony. In response, a gathering of some 3,000 black Philadelphians reaffirmed the commitment of the Free Africans to build a black community and to struggle on behalf of the enslaved. "Our ancestors (not of choice) were the first successful cultivators of the wilds of America," they declared.

> We their descendants feel ourselves entitled to participate in the blessings of her luxuriant soil, with their blood and sweat manured; and that any measure having a tendency to banish us from her bosom, would not

only be cruel, but in direct violation of those principles which have been the boast of this republic. We never will separate ourselves voluntarily from the slave population in this country; they are our brethren by the ties of consanguinity, of suffering, and of wrong.[46]

Again, in 1838, when Pennsylvania adopted a new constitution specifically denying black voting rights, Philadelphia African Americans rose to defend the character of their community, invoking the memory of 1793: "When the yellow fever ravaged Philadelphia and the whites fled, and there were not found enough of them in the city to bury their dead, the colored people volunteered to do that painful and dangerous duty. It is notorious that many whites who were forsaken by their own relations and left to the mercy of this fell disease, were nursed gratuitously by the colored people. Does this speak an enmity which would abuse the privileges of civil liberty to the injury of the whites?"[47]

In the last years of his life Richard Allen wrote his autobiography, finally published in 1833. He was a founder and first Bishop of the first African American religious denomination, and one of the last acts of his ministry was to organize and convene the first national convention of African American leaders. But he wrote of none of that. Instead he told of his life in slavery, first in Philadelphia and later in Delaware, his struggle to work himself free, his call to preach the gospel, and his wandering ministry. He wrote of the formation of the Free African Society and the emergence from it of Bethel Church; and he wrote of the struggles of the men and women of Bethel for their autonomy and their final coming together with other black congregations into the A.M.E. Church. He appended to his life story two documents which he thought were critical for future generations, the African Supplement of the original Bethel charter which sets forth the organizational principles of Bethel's autonomy, and the 1793 *Narrative*. These were new times and, as in our era, blacks had considered the question of what might be a respectable term by which to designate themselves. "Colored" was the common consensus, and "Colored Americans," "men and women of color," "people of color," were preferred terms. Accommodating contemporary sensibilities, Allen changed the text, substituting "colored" for "black."[48]

An account of the humblest portion of his life, the creation of an autonomous black church, and the narrative of 1793 are what Allen chose to pass on to posterity in his autobiography. It was reprinted in at least ten editions, a continuing legacy for Philadelphia African Americans. Fittingly, the legacy continues in the 1993 edition published by the National Park Service in commemoration of the bicentennial of the 1793 epidemic.[49] It is the quintessential artifact of the lives, times, and struggles of the Free Africans and the black Philadelphians of 1793—of Jones, Allen, and Abigail.

NOTES

1. Carey published three editions of his pamphlet between 13 November and 30 November; a fourth edition on 16 January 1794, and reprint editions in the 1830s. For a detailed study of Carey's *Short Account*, see Sally F. Griffith's essay in this volume.

2. Carey, *Short Account of the Malignant Fever, Lately Prevalent in Philadelphia*, 3rd Ed. Improved (Philadelphia: Mathew Carey, 1793), p. 78. Except where noted, quotes from Carey's pamphlet are from this third edition, the last noted by Jones and Allen.

3. Ibid., pp. 33–34.

4. Ibid., p. 78.

5. John H. Powell, *Bring Out Your Dead: The Great Plague of Yellow Fever in Philadelphia in 1793* (Philadelphia: University of Pennsylvania Press, 1949), p. 98.

6. *Minutes of the Proceedings of the Committee . . . to Attend to and Alleviate the Sufferings of the Afflicted with the Malignant Fever, Prevalent, in the City and Its Vicinity, With an Appendix* (Philadelphia: Printed by R. Aitken, 1794). Unnumbered folding tables following p. 204 enumerate fatalities, white and black populations, and the number of those who fled from each group. My numbers are calculated from those areas reporting 75 or more fatalities.

7. Billy G. Smith and Richard Wojtowicz, comps., *Blacks Who Stole Themselves: Advertisements for Runaways in the Pennsylvania Gazette, 1728–1790* (Philadelphia: University of Pennsylvania Press, 1989).

8. *Federal Gazette*, 2 October 1793.

9. Absalom Jones and Richard Allen, *A Narrative of the Proceedings of the Black People, During the Late Awful Calamity in Philadelphia in the Year 1793: And a Refutation of Some Censures, Thrown upon Them in Some Late Publications* (Philadelphia: Printed for the Authors, by William W. Woodward, 1794), pp. 12–13.

10. Ibid., p. 14.

11. William Douglass, *Annals of the First African Church, in the United States of America, Now Styled the African Episcopal Church of St. Thomas* (Philadelphia: King and Baird, 1862), pp. 107–110; Gary B. Nash, *Forging Freedom: The Formation of Philadelphia's Black Community, 1720–1840* (Cambridge: Harvard University Press, 1988), p. 132.

12. Benjamin Rush to Julia Rush, 25 September 1793, in *Letters of Benjamin Rush*, ed. L. H. Butterfield, 2 vols. (Princeton: Princeton University Press, 1951), 2: 684.

13. Carey, *Short Account*, p. 10; *Letters of Benjamin Rush*, 2: 658; Jones and Allen, *Narrative*, p. 8.

14. Jones and Allen, *Narrative*, pp. 6–8, 21–23.

15. John Edgar Wideman, "Fever," in *Fever: Twelve Stories* (New York: Henry Holt, 1989), p. 150.

16. Jones and Allen, *Narrative*, p. 15.

17. *Minutes of the Proceedings of the Committee*, p. 193 (misnumbered as 186).

18. My thanks to social historian and demographer Susan E. Klepp who provided some very useful numbers and analysis. See also Christ Church (Philadelphia), *Mortality. An Account of the Baptisms and Burials from December 25, 1792, to December 25, 1793* [Philadelphia, 1793]; and Klepp's essay in this volume.

19. Jones and Allen, *Narrative*, pp. 11–12; *Minutes of the Proceedings of the Committee*, pp. 185–204.
20. Carey, *Short Account . . . Fourth Edition, Improved* (Philadelphia: Printed by the Author, 1794), p. 121.
21. Materials examined searching for Abigail include: Pennsylvania Abolition Society records of manumissions and indentures, Committee of Guardians minutes, Committee for Improving the Condition of Free Blacks minutes; city directories; 1790 Census; lists of black names in William Douglass, *Annals of the First African Church* (Philadelphia: King and Baird, 1862), with Free African Society minutes and early church members; and Almshouse records at Philadelphia City Archives.
22. Jones and Allen, *Narrative*, p. 15.
23. Richard Folwell, *Short History of the Yellow Fever, That Broke Out in the City of Philadelphia, in July, 1797* (Philadelphia: Printed by Richard Folwell, 1797), p. 23.
24. Jones and Allen, *Narrative*, p. 23.
25. Ibid., pp. 26–28. For similar black admonitions to other blacks see Cyrus Bustill, "An Address to the Blacks in Philadelfiea 9th month 18th 1787," *William and Mary Quarterly*, 3rd ser., 29(1972): 103; and Jupiter Hammon, *An Address to the Negroes, in the State of New York* (New York: Printed; Philadelphia, Reprinted by Daniel Humphreys, 1787). This particular edition of Hammon is a reprint of the New York, 1787, edition, published in an edition of 500 copies and distributed by the Pennsylvania Abolition Society.
26. Jones and Allen, *Narrative*, p. 28.
27. Mathew Carey, *Address of M. Carey to the Public* (Philadelphia: Mathew Carey, 1794), p. 5.
28. *Federal Gazette*, 23 September 1793.
29. W.E.B. Du Bois, *The Philadelphia Negro: A Social Study* (New York: Benjamin Blom, 1965), p. 19.
30. Surviving minutes of the Free African Society are in William Douglass, *Annals of the First African Church*. For a good analysis of Philadelphia black life in this time, see Nash, *Forging Freedom*; and Julie Winch, *Philadelphia's Black Elite: Activism, Accommodation, and the Struggle for Autonomy, 1787–1848* (Philadelphia: Temple University Press, 1988), particularly chapter 1.
31. Ira V. Brown, "Pennsylvania's Antislavery Pioneers, 1688–1776," *Pennsylvania History* 55 (1988): 69–70.
32. *American Weekly Mercury*, 5 February 1723.
33. John C. Van Horne, ed., *Religious Philanthropy and Colonial Slavery: The American Correspondence of the Associates of Dr. Bray, 1717–1777* (Urbana and Chicago: University of Illinois Press, 1985), p. 23.
34. James Hardie, *The Philadelphia Directory and Register* (Philadelphia: T. Dobson, 1793), p. 199.
35. There is no readily available single source for the activities of the PAS. However, their activities and relations with blacks are well presented in Nash, *Forging Freedom*.
36. See Gary B. Nash and Jean R. Soderlund, *Freedom By Degrees: Emancipation in Pennsylvania and Its Aftermath* (New York: Oxford University Press, 1991), particularly chapter 5.
37. See, for example, Ferdinando Fairfax, "Plan for Liberating the Negroes Within

the United States," *American Museum* 8 (1790): 285; and Jonathan Edwards, *The Injustice and Impolicy of the Slave Trade* (New Haven: Printed by Thomas and Samuel Green, 1791), pp. 34–37.

38. William Douglass, *Annals*, p. 28.

39. *Encyclopaedia; or, a Dictionary of Arts, Sciences and Miscellaneous Literature* (Philadelphia: Thomas Dobson, 1798), 10:794–799, see entry for "Negro."

40. Richard Allen, *Life, Experience and Gospel Labours* (Philadelphia: Martin and Boden, Printers, 1833), p. 13. There is some confusion over dating this event. In *The Doctrines and Discipline of the African Methodist Episcopal Church* (Philadelphia: John H. Cunningham, 1817), Allen dates it as 1787. However, in his autobiography he is not specific, and clearly telescopes events of several years into a quick summary. He does, however, mention blacks being confined to a gallery. An examination of St. George's records reveals this gallery did not exist until around June, 1792. See Nash, *Forging Freedom*, p. 310 (n. 62) for a summary discussion. However, I am not entirely convinced that the evidence dating the gallery construction invalidates Allen's date. I think it unlikely that Allen, hardly in his dotage in 1817, would have mislaid five years. Perhaps the later construction of the gallery to which blacks were to be restricted might have, years later, merged with the original event in Allen's mind as a metaphor for being cast out.

41. Sidney Kaplan, *The Black Presence in the Era of the American Revolution, 1770–1800* (New York: New York Graphic Society Ltd. and Smithsonian Institution Press, 1973), pp. 231–240. On kidnapping, see [Edward Darlington], *Reflections on Slavery; With Recent Evidence of Its Inhumanity . . . By Humanitas* (Philadelphia: For the Author by R. Cochran, 1803); Jesse Torrey, *A Portraiture of Domestic Slavery, in the United States* (Philadelphia: Published by the Author, John Bioren, Printer, 1817); and a summary study, Julie Winch, "Philadelphia and the Other Underground Railroad," *Pennsylvania Magazine of History and Biography* 111 (1987): 3–25.

42. *Register of Pennsylvania*, 12 March 1831, p. 163 enumerates 44 black organizations founded since the 1790s. The list is not definitive.

43. *Dictionary of American Negro Biography* (New York and London: W.W. Norton, 1982), pp. 12, 234, 362.

44. [Joseph Willson], *Sketches of the Higher Classes of Colored Society in Philadelphia* (Philadelphia: Merrihew and Thompson, 1841), p. 101.

45. Prince Saunders, *An Address, Delivered at Bethel Church, Philadelphia . . . Before the Pennsylvania Augustinian Society, for the Education of People of Colour* (Philadelphia: Joseph Rakestraw, 1818); Winch, *Philadelphia's Black Elite*, chapter 2. Many of these old Philadelphia-Haitian families are still there. We occasionally meet their younger generations at the Library Company, where they come to research these early movements and their black Philadelphia heritage.

46. *Poulson's American Daily Advertiser*, 11 August 1817.

47. Robert Purvis, *Appeal of Forty Thousand Citizens, Threatened with Dis-Franchisement, to the People of Pennsylvania* (Philadelphia: Merrihew and Gunn, 1838), pp. 11, 14.

48. Richard Allen, *Life, Experiences and Gospel Labours*, wherein the 1794 work is retitled *Narrative of the Proceedings of the Coloured People*.

49. Powell, *Bring Out Your Dead*.

Passions and Politics:
The Multiple Meanings of Benjamin
Rush's Treatment for Yellow Fever

JACQUELYN C. MILLER

N 19 August 1793, two of Benjamin Rush's medical colleagues, Dr. Hugh Hodge and Dr. John Foulke, requested his presence at the Philadelphia home of French importer Peter LeMaigre at 77 Water Street. Hodge and Foulke sought Rush's advice regarding the treatment of Catherine LeMaigre, Peter's thirty-three-year-old wife, who was not only suffering from an intense burning heat in her stomach but was also constantly vomiting a black bile. Though Rush was unable at that time to offer any lifesaving remedy for his fevered patient, who died the following evening, the ensuing exchange of information with his peers enabled Rush to name the disease that had lately killed a number of his patients. It was in the LeMaigres' parlor, then, that Rush first announced that Philadelphia was in the midst of a major outbreak of yellow fever, its fifth in ninety-four years.[1]

Rush's name, more than any other, is synonymous with the epidemic of 1793. This indelible linkage of man and event has largely been the result of the intense controversy surrounding Rush's infamous method of treating yellow fever with an aggressive regimen of mercurial purging and profuse, or in Rush's words, "copious bloodletting."[2] In September of that year, in a letter to the College of Physicians of Philadelphia, he said, "I consider intrepidity in the use of the lancet at present to be as necessary as it is in the use of mercury and jalap in this insidious and ferocious disease."[3] The boldness of Rush's therapy, in which he advocated in extreme cases the loss of up to four-fifths of the blood in the body, was partly the result of his conviction that the magnitude of the crisis called for drastic measures. But, as I argue in this essay, more was at stake than just the lives of the fever's victims or Rush's professional reputation. Rush was passionately involved in the creation of state and federal constitutions during the post-Revolutionary period. In addition, he was vitally interested in both the moral and the physical constitutions of the individuals for whom those documents were devised. Consequently, his medical treat-

79

ments were infused with important social and political meanings that historians have largely overlooked.[4]

Rush believed that "order and tranquillity" in the body politic depended on the existence of "a well-balanced republic"; analogously, his idea of a healthy body also emphasized the need for equilibrium, which was to be maintained through a combination of dietary, hygienic, environmental, physical, and medical means. Thus, just as Rush anticipated that frequent elections would release the social and political tension built up among competing factions within the body politic, so he expected that purging and bleeding would remove the surplus of stimulus from the physical system and would relieve the vascular pressures that resulted when the body was in a diseased state. The ramifications of Rush's treatment for yellow fever, then, were not solely medical. Instead, because yellow fever was only one of a long list of "pestilences" that Rush encountered during the post-war period—including scourges of mob violence, democratic impulses, intemperance, and vice—his reaction to the epidemic is best understood within the context of his larger social and political concerns. Or, more precisely, his response should be envisioned as a struggle to avert a second American Revolution, a conflict he dreaded might lead to a reign of terror comparable to the one underway in France.

Late in the evening two very busy days after he had encountered his first case of yellow fever, Rush, though physically exhausted and low in spirits, sat down to write his wife, Julia, about the malignant fever that had broken out in Water Street between Arch and Race Streets. He anxiously reported to Julia, who had been visiting her parents in Princeton for some weeks, that he had lost three patients to the fever out of the 12 or so persons who had fallen victim, while attending another seven or eight who had survived.[5] In his next letter, four days later, Rush painted an even grimmer picture of health conditions in Philadelphia, relating how the fever "not only mocks in most instances the power of medicine, but it has spread through several parts of the city remote from the spot where it originated." The area where the disease had first struck was "nearly desolated by it," and the dreadful scenes he witnessed while carrying out his professional duties reminded him of stories he had read of the plague, particularly the speed with which huge numbers of people were dying. Rush recounted how two of his patients had succumbed to the disease the night before, while "five other persons died in the neighborhood yesterday afternoon and four more last night at Kensington."[6] As evidenced by his correspondence with Julia and by his later recollection that "heaven alone bore witness to the anguish of my soul in this awful situation," Rush obviously suffered a great deal of frustration and sorrow over his inability to save the victims of the fever.[7]

Rush, however, was always one to maintain a modicum of optimism, even

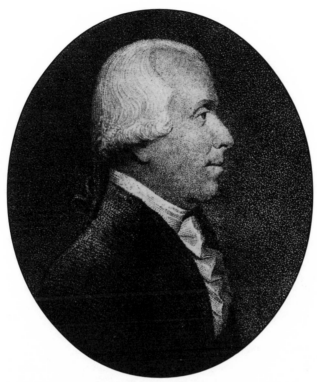

Benjamin Rush, from an engraving in the *American Universal Magazine*, n.d. Courtesy of the Library of the College of Physicians of Philadelphia.

during life's darkest moments.[8] Despite the fact that by the third week of the epidemic he had tried all the common remedies with little or no success, he, working from the assumption that "there does not exist a disease for which the goodness of Providence has not provided a remedy," continued to confer with other physicians and to pore over every book in his library that dealt with the subject of yellow fever. Such was his fervent desire to find a medical treatment that would alleviate the pain and despair of his suffering patients and their families.[9] According to Rush's description of his actions during these early weeks of the epidemic, his persistence soon paid off. Within the week he had rediscovered in his possession "a manuscript account of the yellow fever as it prevailed in Virginia in the year 1741, which had been put into my hands by Dr. Franklin a short time before his death."[10] It was this document that led Rush to develop his new method of treating the fever, a treatment he soon touted as no less than a miracle cure.[11] Almost from the first moment, however, when Rush began to give his patients massive doses of purgatives containing equal measures of calomel and jalap and to bleed them profusely, his intrepid regimen became a topic of acute scrutiny and fierce controversy among his contemporaries, and a subject that has intrigued historians for nearly a century.[12]

In recent decades Rush's method of treatment has been attacked, explained, or defended by scholars from a variety of positions. For instance, Victor Robinson, from a stance of twentieth-century hindsight, but sounding very much like Rush's most ardent eighteenth-century detractors, has severely criticized Rush's proclivity for mercury and the lancet by deriding him for "his paucity of thought," and calling him a "menace in the sick-room."[13] Other historians, including J. H. Powell, while evaluating Rush's adherence to heroic measures in less disparaging terms, have nevertheless puzzled over and attempted to explain how "the brilliant Benjamin Rush [could] have come to believe as he did, and with egregious obstinacy stick to his belief."[14] In their view it was Rush's flawed character that allowed him "to discard every canon of scientific caution, and in one week to proclaim desperate remedies a new principle in medicine."[15]

A few attempts, however, have been made to understand Rush's propensity for a vigorous interventionist method from the perspective of eighteenth-century medical knowledge, pointing out that even though Rush's treatment was extreme, the reasoning behind it was nonetheless sound.[16] Richard Shryock, for example, emphasized the fact that Rush's medical system drew to a great extent upon the pathologic theories of his teacher William Cullen and of his fellow student John Brown, while Chris Holmes defended Rush's therapy as the "product of contemplation and logical thinking."[17] While these works make a good case for understanding how Rush reached the conclusions he did in terms of contemporary medical concepts, they fail to explain adequately why Rush rejected the more complex theories of disease advanced by Cullen and Brown or why the use of such strong measures to treat the fever made so much sense to him. In order to discover what contributed to Rush's theories and practices regarding disease and health, it is necessary to look beyond the medical world as these scholars have narrowly defined it. Also, by extending our analysis chronologically to the two decades preceding the yellow fever epidemic, we are better able to apprehend the main course of Rush's development.

Rush was only one of many writers of his generation who assumed that the organization of social and political systems and the health of the people who populated those systems were so mutually related that any widespread modifications in social relationships would produce accompanying changes in the health of the people involved. According to medical historian George Rosen,

Rush, along with Thomas Jefferson, presented the most precisely expressed opinions on the subject.[18] One of Rush's clearest, as well as earliest, statements on this topic is in his *Inquiry into the Natural History of Medicine Among the Indians of North America*, which he read before the American Philosophical Society on 4 February 1774.[19] According to Rush,

> the abolition of the feudal system in Europe, by introducing freedom, introduced at the same time agriculture; which by multiplying the fruits of the earth, lessened the consumption of animal food, and thus put a stop to [leprosy, elephantiasis, scurvy, venereal disease, plica polonica, smallpox, and the plague].[20]

In Rush's opinion, then, an awareness of the interrelatedness of political slavery and particular diseases that deform and debase the human body could only serve as a powerful motive "to enhance the blessings of liberty [and] to trace its effects in eradicating such loathsome and destructive disorders."[21] The description of Rush's commitment to liberty that is laid out in the following pages should thus be viewed in light of his concerns regarding health and social welfare issues.

The local political conflicts of the late 1770s brought Rush's attention close to home. In contrast to what he called the "mob government" that had been constituted in 1776, Rush argued that Pennsylvania's previous government was one of the happiest in the world, and that "nothing more was necessary to have made us a free and happy people than to abolish the royal and proprietary power of the state."[22] The democratical tendencies of the Constitution of 1776, Rush argued, went much too far in the other direction, exposing its citizens to all the miseries of tyranny and licentiousness without providing a "remedy" for either.[23]

For Rush, then, the Pennsylvania Constitution symbolized a consequence of the struggle for independence that he had not anticipated—the increased interest and involvement of people who had previously played little role in the political process. He was forced to acknowledge their presence time and time again, not only as a result of the controversies that continued to surround the creation of state and federal governments, but also by other actions that the common folk took in order to make their voices heard.[24] But he did not welcome their participation. Instead, he viewed their involvement as potentially dangerous and preferred that members of the lower classes not discuss politics at all, remarking once that the less servants argued over political subjects the better, as "such disputes, especially among ignorant people, generally confirm prejudices and increase obstinacy."[25] Underlying this elitist view of politics was a definite fear that popular politics would encourage social disorder, and, hence, would foster an outbreak of violence.[26]

Rush's reaction to the Fort Wilson incident demonstrates very clearly his growing intolerance of civil disorder of any kind. According to historian Robert Brunhouse, the afternoon battle that occurred at the house of former Congressman James Wilson on 4 October 1779, between a group of poor militiamen and several "gentlemen" who were ostensibly guarding the property, was "the highwater mark of radical democracy in Pennsylvania during the revolutionary period."[27] The incident, which resulted in an estimated six or seven deaths and more than twice that number wounded, began as a demonstration by the soldiers who protested having to shoulder an unequal share of the war's military and economic burdens.[28] Rush's response to the conflict made it apparent that his sympathies lay with the gentlemen, particularly Colonel Wilson "whose only crime was having pled in some cases for the tories." On the other hand, Rush expressed little concern for the plight of the militiamen, remarking that "the objects of the mob were unknown or confusedly understood"; he focused instead on the fact that "our streets were for the first time stained with fraternal blood."[29] The event, in Rush's opinion, was proof that "Poor Pennsylvania" had degenerated from a democracy to a mobocracy and had, consequently, become "the most miserable spot upon the surface of the globe."[30]

Regardless of Rush's gloomy assessment of Pennsylvania's social and political well-being following the Fort Wilson episode, his mood, as revealed in his writings, was in constant flux throughout the decade, vacillating between a sense of pessimism and optimism, depending on whether the turn of events seemed to be going his way.[31] And Rush continued to believe during this period that the primary treatment for the disorder that was afflicting the body politic was a properly balanced system of government.[32] This assumption led him to declare a few years later that "I have pledged myself to my friends that I will never relinquish the great object of a good constitution."[33]

Despite Rush's anticipation that the new federal Constitution of 1787, "like a new continental wagon," would "overset our state dung cart with all its dirty contents," and, therefore, provide the perfect vehicle for "traveling fast into order and national happiness," it became increasingly clear by the early 1790s that new governments in and of themselves would not bring about the social stability and harmony he desired so much.[34] Of course, Rush had never rested his hopes totally on the creation of a particular political system. Even during the very early years of the independence movement, Rush had initiated a parallel campaign to "effect a revolution in our principles, opinions, and manners so as to accommodate them to the forms of government we have adopted."[35] Rush's constitutional concerns thus had long had a dual dimension. While as a physician he had always been concerned with the well-being of the physical body, his energies in the 1780s were focused to a great extent on the health of political constitutions. By the 1790s, however, when Rush turned his efforts more decidedly toward the treatment of biological constitutions, the social struggles of the previous decade caused him to think of his patients' bodies as political, as well as physical, entities.[36]

Rush frequently portrayed the lower classes as being ruled entirely by their passions. But he often went even further. In a lecture on "Diseases of the Passions," which he gave at the University of Pennsylvania sometime before 1792, Rush also associated with the passions the political representatives of those members of society who make up the "body" of the body politic.[37] According to Rush, "the human mind may be compared to the British government."

> The Will is the King; the Understanding, the House of Lords; the Passions, the House of Commons; the Moral Faculty, the Court of Westminster; and the Conscience, the High Court of Chancery.
>
> To this last are all appeals made, it is above all Law and answerable only to the Supreme Being.
>
> As the Government can be well conducted only when these five powers harmonize with each other, so the Mind can alone act equably and right when the Harmony of its Powers is perfect.[38]

Given Rush's tendency to link unleashed passions with the non-ruling classes, it is not surprising that he considered the House of Commons "the most turbulent and most liable to disturbance and corruption of any part of the British Government," and "in the same manner are the Passions most liable to be misled and become turbulent."[39] Rush's analysis, then, implicitly connected the passions with the masses, whereas the will, the conscience, the moral sense, and reason were associated with the elite members of society. He recognized that "notwithstanding all, the Passions are an important part of the Mind, and are not without their use."[40] But even this backhanded compliment carried with it an insult given that Rush judged the masses to be of little worth in and of themselves. They became valuable only when they were useful to, and therefore a *part* of, the sphere of the ruling classes.

One way Rush thought the passions of the people often became inflamed was through the continued use of alcoholic beverages. For instance, he blamed the riot at Fort Wilson on the unsubstantiated assumption that the soldiers were "enraged chiefly by liquor."[41] Beyond specific associations of alcohol with social disorder and violence, Rush also metaphorically connected spirituous liquors and lower class involvement in political affairs. For example, he attributed the democratic tendencies of the Pennsylvania Constitution of 1776, a document that was largely the work of new men in government with a decidedly radical agenda, to the people being "intoxicated" with the "first flowing of liberty," while complaining that "all our laws breathe the spirit of town meetings and porter shops."[42]

While gentlemen were the intended constituency for Rush's first public and implicitly political pronouncements advocating temperance in the early 1770s, he widened his audience considerably by the end of the century.[43] By this time he had also built quite an elaborate case against drinking spirituous liquors, based on their major role in causing physical, moral, and political disorder. In his 1772 *Sermons to Gentlemen* Rush argued that wine or strong drink may be given to the sick, inhabitants of low marshy countries, and to old people, but should not be given to children, studious people, or young people.[44] In this account Rush did assert that there is an "inseparable connection between intemperance and disease," though given his audience, it is not surprising that the only disease he discussed was gout.[45]

Around 1784 Rush published his most extensive argument to date against using spirituous liquors, proposing for the first time that alcohol is a cause of vice and tracing the negative effect drinking could have on a society as a whole. While Rush admitted that "a strong constitution, especially if it be assisted with constant and hard labor, will counteract the destructive effects of spirits for many years," he nevertheless blamed alcohol for causing many disorders, including a sickness in the stomach, a universal dropsy, obstruction of the liver, pains in the limbs, epilepsy, madness, palsy, and apoplexy. Rush also maintained that intemperance could have profound social and political ramifications, since

> a people corrupted with strong drink cannot long be a *free* people. The rulers of such a community will soon partake of the vices of that mass from which they were secreted, and all our laws and governments will sooner or later bear the same marks of the effects of spirituous liquors which were described formerly upon individuals.[46]

While this statement was contemporary with Rush's comments comparing the human mind to the British government, it nevertheless suggests an additional concern that Rush had regarding the use of alcohol. His view that rulers would be influenced by the vices of the people reveals a fear that liquor worked to reverse or to hinder the proper functioning of society just as it did that of the body, while also intimating that the head of the body politic was susceptible to contamination by the drinking masses.

The existence of a vital conceptual link between Rush's political views and his ideas about disease is particularly apparent in his 1789 essay on the effects of the military and political events of the American Revolution on the human body.[47] According to Rush, since the minds of the citizens of the United States were wholly unprepared for peace in 1783, "the excess of the passion for liberty, inflamed by the successful issue of the war, produced, in many people opinions and conduct which could not be removed by reason nor restrained by government." As a result, he believed that "the extensive influence which these opinions had upon the understandings, passions and morals of many of the citizens" constituted a species of insanity he named *Anarchia*.[48] Rush's interpretation reflected the assumptions advanced in the popular medical literature of the time, particularly the belief that expressions of violent passion resulted in temporary madness. And Rush increasingly came to see madness as a disease that could be treated like any other.[49]

Rush contended in his discussion of the moral faculty that disease, like other physical conditions, could also have a negative effect on one's ability to choose between good and evil. While he believed that fevers and madness most frequently disposed one to vice, he also thought that hysteria and hypochondriasis, as well as other states of the body "accompanied with preternatural irritability, sensibility, torpor, stupor, or mobility of the nervous system," could contribute to immoral behavior. Because the moral faculty in these situations was impaired as the result of disease, Rush suggested a medical regimen consisting of exercise, the cold bath, and a change in the atmosphere.[50] Clearly, then, by the 1790s Rush had expanded the physician's purview to cover the realms of moral and mental illness, areas that had also been affected by the larger political and social struggles of the Revolutionary era.

Rush began the final decade of the eighteenth century with a dream that it would be less politically turbulent than the previous twenty years had been. Expressing this hope to John Adams in 1790, Rush wrote that "the peaceable manner in which our constitutions have been changed in the United States and in Pennsylvania make it probable that man is becoming a more rational creature in America than in other parts of the world."[51] And since in a "well-balanced republic . . . men can remove the evils of their governments by frequent elections, they will seldom appeal to the less certain remedies of mobs or arms," thereby assuring that "order and tranquility" are the "natural consequence" of a correctly constituted political system.[52] Rush also had high expectations regarding the physical health of the country, since he believed that "passions produce fewer diseases in a republic than in a monarchy," and that in time "the effects of the political passions upon health and life will be still less perceptible in our country."[53] But as Rush soon learned, following the onset of the French Revolution, politics in the 1790s was to become even more passionate, uncontrollable even by the strictures of the newly created constitutions.[54]

As he had done in 1779 following the battle at Fort Wilson, Rush continued to consider the lower classes' tendency toward disorder and violence potentially life-threatening in more ways than one, especially considering that the new constitutions were proving to be ineffectual as preventive measures.[55] While bloodshed was a potential consequence of most crowd actions, Rush's belief that the agitated state of politics in general, which was a result of people's inability or unwillingness to control their physical passions, and could also cause death through disease, had important implications for the medical theories and regimen he developed during the yellow fever epidemic in 1793.[56]

Rush's assumptions concerning the issues of health and disease suggest that he consciously devised his regimen of aggressive bloodletting and intense purging as a means of controlling the passions of the body politic.[57] His expectation that moral, political, and physical health were all dependent upon one another, revealed in his tendency to use political metaphors when talking about the body and medical and disease images when discussing issues of a political nature, would have led him to such a conclusion. Also, Rush's reduction of the more complicated theories of disease promoted by his colleagues William Cullen and John Brown to his own view that all illness was "a form of morbid excitement" produced by an overstimulation of the whole system, reflected his preoccupation with the excesses of the members of the body politic as a result of the American Revolution.[58] Therefore, it makes sense to argue that he was aware that his efforts to treat yellow fever in 1793 had a significance beyond the medical sphere.

Technically, then, the disorder Rush treated in 1793 was not merely yellow fever, but was an inflammatory action in the system, which was the consequence of an overabundance of stimuli. Rush's unitary theory of disease is also more understandable if examined in light of his intense yearning for social harmony and his concomitant anxiety over the continuing existence of political factions and social fragmentation. And his insistence that the yellow fever had chased all other diseases from the city, making it a "monarchical disorder," can be viewed as an effort to unite Philadelphians once again to oppose a common enemy.[59]

But when it became clear to Rush in the 1790s that balanced constitutions and recurrent elections had failed to achieve their appropriate ends, he took matters even further into his own hands. Rush's belief that all disease was the product of capillary stress, and thus necessitated depleting remedies, guaranteed, in his mind, that large numbers of overstimulated bodies could eventually be calmed through a regimen of bleeding and purging. Thus, blood would be shed in America as in France, but the indiscriminate flowing of blood unleashed by the French Reign of Terror would be replaced in America by a set of controlled conditions in which bloodletting would be practiced under the close supervision of a trained expert and only on the diseased elements of the political body.

During the 1790s Rush never openly linked the social and political implications of his purging and bleeding regimen, but he did so several years later. Writing to John Adams in 1806, Rush disclosed a great antipathy toward the country's leaders in his proposal that the remedies for a yellow fever would do wonders with the heads of the men who now move our world. Ten and ten (as our doses of calomel and jalap were called in 1793) would be a substitute for a fistula in the bowels of Bonaparte. Bleeding would probably lessen the rage for altering the Constitution of Pennsylvania in the leaders of the party who are now contending for that measure. Tonics might be useful to those persons who behold with timidity the insults and spoliations that are offered to our commerce. The cold bath might cure the peevish irritability of some of the members of our Congress, and blisters and mustard plasters rouse the apathy of others. In short, there is a great field opened for new means of curing moral and political maladies.[60]

Even at the ripe old age of sixty, Rush continued to view the world of politics through the mind of a physician and to address medical concerns in light of their impact on the body politic. It is not surprising then, that, in addition to its purpose as a medical regimen, Rush's controversial treatment for yellow fever was also a technique to control the passions of the country's inhabitants, particularly the lower classes.[61] By the time of the yellow fever epidemic of 1793, Rush believed that if those members of society who constituted an arm, a leg, or the belly of the body politic were pacified, the masses would no longer attempt to usurp the functions of the governing head. Achieving command over the passions would result in a healthy body politic where people of all classes, colors, and creeds could live together in virtuous accord. Rush's effort to achieve his utopian dream, however, not only put his medical reputation in jeopardy, but reveals a strand of social conservatism that has largely gone unexplored.

NOTES

1. Benjamin Rush, *An Account of the Bilious Remitting Yellow Fever, as It Appeared in the City of Philadelphia, in the Year 1793* (Philadelphia: Thomas Dobson, 1794), pp. 11–13; Rush to Julia Rush, 21 August 1793, *Letters of Benjamin Rush*, ed. L. H. Butterfield, 2 vols. (Princeton, N.J.: Princeton University Press, 1951), 2: 637; and J. H. Powell, *Bring Out Your Dead: The Great Plague of Yellow Fever in Philadelphia in 1793* (Philadelphia: University of Pennsylvania Press, 1949; reprint, New York: Time Incorporated, 1965, and Philadelphia: University of Pennsylvania Press, 1993), pp. 11–12.

2. Rush, *Account*, pp. 200–204, 271; Rush to John R. B. Rodgers, 3 October 1793, *Letters*, 2: 695; and Carl Binger, *Revolutionary Doctor: Benjamin Rush, 1746–1813* (New York: W. W. Norton and Co., 1966), p. 228.

3. Rush to the College of Physicians of Philadelphia, 12 September 1793, *Letters*, 2: 661.

4. I have reviewed the limitations of the historiography dealing with Rush's controversial treatment of yellow fever later in the text in an effort to situate my study

within that rather large body of literature. Although I argue throughout this essay that in order to understand Rush on his own terms we must broaden our scope of analysis to the social and political conflicts of his day, it is important to note that I am not the first to do so. For example, Martin S. Pernick reminded us over twenty years ago that "political fears could easily distort medical objectivity." See his "Politics, Parties, and Pestilence: Epidemic Yellow Fever in Philadelphia and the Rise of the First Party System," reprinted in this volume (quote on p. 125). Pernick's contribution to the social history of medicine has thus been significant, though his statistical evidence is certainly somewhat debatable and, as the remainder of my essay reveals, his characterization of Rush as a democrat is quite suspect (p. 129). Nevertheless, my work builds on Pernick's in that I have applied his insights into the world of party politics in the 1790s to the broader realm of eighteenth-century political culture in order to study the values and assumptions that lay behind Rush's medical beliefs and practices.

5. Rush to Julia Rush, 21 August 1793, *Old Family Letters Relating to the Yellow Fever*, Series B (Philadelphia: J. B. Lippincott Company, 1892), p. 3.

6. Rush to Julia Rush, 25 August 1793, ibid., p. 5.

7. Rush, *Account*, p. 196.

8. George Rosen, "Political Order and Human Health in Jeffersonian Thought," *Bulletin of the History of Medicine* 26 (1952): 35–36.

9. For Rush's version of his quest for a cure, see his *Account*, pp. 193–204; quote from page 196.

10. Ibid., p. 197. Dr. John Mitchell (d. 1768) of Virginia was the author of this manuscript, which was actually a 1744 letter to Cadwallader Colden. The letter was published, in part, in the *Philadelphia Medical Museum* 1 (1805): 1–21, and in its entirety in the *American Medical and Philosophical Register* 4 (1814): 181–215. For additional information regarding this document, see *Letters of Benjamin Rush*, 2: 700, n. 10; *The Papers of Benjamin Franklin*, ed. Leonard W. Labaree, et al. (New Haven: Yale University Press, 1959–), 3: 17–21, 41–44; and Saul Jarcho, "John Mitchell, Benjamin Rush, and Yellow Fever," *Bulletin of the History of Medicine* 31 (1957): 132–36. Jarcho argued that at least five of the six cases that Mitchell reported were not yellow fever.

11. The section of the manuscript that had the greatest impact on Rush's treatment was Mitchell's statement that he did not hesitate to give purges to his patients who suffered from acute putrid fevers, even when their pulse rate was so low that he could hardly feel it. He argued that the evacuations were necessary in order to bring the fever "to a perfect crisis, and solution." See Rush's *Account*, p. 198. At least one historian has mistakenly credited Mitchell with promoting bleeding in addition to purging as a treatment for yellow fever (see Chris Holmes, "Benjamin Rush and the Yellow Fever," *Bulletin of the History of Medicine* 40 (1966): 249.) For an example of Rush's high opinion of his new treatment, see his *Account*, p. 204.

12. Though Rush's regimen had many contemporary critics, an aggressive approach to treating disease, known as "heroic therapeutics," became very widespread in the early decades of the nineteenth century, but declined in popularity by mid-century. For accounts of the contemporary debates over Rush's treatment, see Powell, *Bring Out Your Dead*, pp. 82–132; William S. Middleton, "The Yellow Fever Epidemic of

1793 in Philadelphia," *Annals of Medical History* 10 (1928): 441–44; Joseph McFarland, "The Epidemic of Yellow Fever in Philadelphia in 1793 and Its Influence Upon Dr. Benjamin Rush," *Medical Life* 36 (1929): 480–96; and Pernick, "Politics, Parties, and Pestilence," pp. 127–130, below. Concerning the impact of Rush's "heroic therapeutics," see Alex Berman, "The Heroic Approach in Nineteenth-Century Therapeutics," *Bulletin of the American Society of Hospital Pharmacists* (1954): 321–27; Charles E. Rosenberg, "The Therapeutic Revolution: Medicine, Meaning, and Social Change in 19th-Century America," in *Sickness and Health in America: Readings in the History of Medicine and Public Health*, 2nd ed., rev., ed. Judith Walzer Leavitt and Ronald L. Numbers (Madison: University of Wisconsin Press, 1985), pp. 46–48; and Joseph Ioor Waring, "The Influence of Benjamin Rush on the Practice of Bleeding in South Carolina," *Bulletin of the History of Medicine* 35 (1961): 230–37. For discussion of Rush's therapeutics in the context of an eighteenth-century understanding of yellow fever, see J. Worth Estes' essay in this volume.

13. Victor Robinson, "The Myth of Benjamin Rush," *Medical Life* 36 (1929): 447–48.

14. Powell, *Bring Out Your Dead*, p. 130.

15. Ibid., p. 131. Joseph McFarland, "Epidemic of Yellow Fever," also focused on character issues to explain Rush's dedication to his method of treatment. In his view, Rush seemed "to have been a man hasty in judgment, obstinate, domineering, bellicose, and overwhelmed by the sense of his own importance" (p. 496). See also Jarcho, "John Mitchell, Benjamin Rush, and Yellow Fever," pp. 132–36.

16. Richard Harrison Shryock, *Medicine and Society in America, 1660–1860* (Ithaca, N.Y.: Great Seal Books, 1960), pp. 58–76; Holmes, "Benjamin Rush and the Yellow Fever," pp. 246–63; and Binger, *Revolutionary Doctor*, pp. 214–16. See also J. Worth Estes' essay in this volume.

17. Shryock, *Medicine and Society*, pp. 68–70; Holmes, "Rush and the Yellow Fever," p. 254.

18. Rosen, "Political Order," p. 32.

19. Rush, "An Inquiry into the Natural History of Medicine Among the Indians of North-America, and a Comparative View of Their Diseases and Remedies, with Those of Civilized Nations," *Medical Inquiries and Observations*, 2nd American ed. (Philadelphia: Thomas Dobson, 1794), 1: 9–77.

20. Ibid., pp. 24–25.

21. Ibid., p. 25.

22. Rush to Anthony Wayne, 19 May 17[77], *Letters*, 1: 148.

23. Rush to John Adams, 12 October 1779, *Letters*, 1: 240.

24. For a discussion of these controversies on a larger scale, see Gordon S. Wood, *The Creation of the American Republic, 1776–1787* (Chapel Hill: University of North Carolina Press, 1969), pp. 393–467. Wood, however, ends his book in 1787 with an account of the creation of the Federal Constitution. But since during the Revolutionary period the word "constitution" meant both a political organization and a bodily condition, efforts to construct an American constitution were not confined to the creation of a new system of government. Rush, for example, focused his energies on improving the health of both the political system and the people who actually embodied it.

25. Rush to Julia Rush, 14 April 1777, *Letters*, 1: 138. The other side of Rush's dissat-

isfaction, however, was his criticism of government officials, military officers, and community leaders who abused their positions of power by failing to act responsibly and selflessly. He believed that if these men lived virtuously and treated the citizenry in a manner not unlike "the conduct of the British Parliament towards the town of Boston in 1774," the lower classes would not have felt the need to demand a say in the political process. See Rush to John Adams, 8 August 1777 and 19 October 1779, *Letters*, 1: 152, 241; Rush (under his Leonidas pseudonym), "A Speech Which Ought to Be Spoken to Congress on the Subject of Inflation," *Pennsylvania Packet*, 3 July 1779; Rush to John Montgomery, 27 June and 4 July 1783, *Letters*, 1: 301, 305.

26. Susan Sontag, in *Illness as Metaphor* (New York: Farrar, Straus and Giroux, 1978), pp. 80–82, has argued that during the late eighteenth century a dramatic change occurred in the metaphorical usage of disease concepts with regard to political ideology, a change she sees as a direct result of the violence of the American and French revolutions. Whereas the republican rhetoric of early-eighteenth-century America stressed the organic nature of social relations inherent in the body politic, and often used disease metaphors to describe social tensions, the tenor of the language made it clear that such friction was not perceived as threatening. As political factionalism and social fragmentation increased during the century, however, the disease metaphors used to describe these new social dynamics took on a more ominous tone, thereby signaling a growing sensitivity to social disorder. While Sontag's work is extremely short on documentation, her argument is borne out by Dorinda Outram in her *The Body and the French Revolution: Sex, Class and Political Culture* (New Haven and London: Yale University Press, 1989), especially chapter 4.

   Rush's writings are a marvelous source for studying this process. I have already mentioned how Rush defined the term "constitution" in two ways. Several other words, including "disorder," also carried multiple meanings.

   For discussions of how disease concepts have been used to construct class and racial identities, see Roy Porter, "Gout: Framing and Fantasizing Diseases," *Bulletin of the History of Medicine* 68 (1994): 1–28; and Joyce E. Chaplin, "Acquired Resistance to Fevers as Cultural Metaphor in Coastal South Carolina and Georgia, 1760–1815" (unpublished manuscript).

27. Robert L. Brunhouse, *The Counter-Revolution in Pennsylvania, 1776–1790* (Harrisburg: Pennsylvania Historical Commission, 1942), p. 75. For a fuller account of the Fort Wilson incident, see Steven Rosswurm, *Arms, Country, and Class: The Philadelphia Militia and the "Lower Sort" During the American Revolution, 1775–1783* (New Brunswick: Rutgers University Press, 1987), pp. 205–227; John K. Alexander, "The Fort Wilson Incident of 1779: A Case Study of the Revolutionary Crowd," *William and Mary Quarterly*, 3rd ser., 31 (1974): 589–612; and C. Page Smith, "The Attack on Fort Wilson," *Pennsylvania Magazine of History and Biography* 78 (1954): 177–88.

28. Rosswurm, *Arms, Country, and Class*, pp. 207–17.

29. Rush to John Adams, 12 October 1779, *Letters*, 1: 240.

30. Rush to Charles Lee, 24 October 1779, *Letters*, 1: 244.

31. Like many of his contemporaries, Rush tended to be more optimistic in his public writings and in his correspondence with Europeans. See Rush, "Citizens of

Pennsylvania of German Birth and Extraction: Proposal of a German College," *Pennsylvania Gazette*, 31 August 1785; Rush to Charles Nesbit, 5 December 1783; 27 April 1784; and 28 November 1784, *Letters*, 1: 316, 330, 344; and Gilbert Chinard, "Eighteenth Century Theories on America as a Human Habitat," *Proceedings of the American Philosophical Society* 91 (1947): 45–52.

32. Rush wrote John Adams in 1789 that a republic was a "government consisting of *three* branches," with each branch being derived "at different times and from different periods from the People." He further added that "where the circulation is wanting between rulers and the ruled, there will be an obstruction to genuine government. A king or a senate not chosen by the people . . . becomes a sebimus, a bubo, or an abscess in the body politic which must sooner or later destroy the healthiest state." On the other hand, "a simple democracy, or an unbalanced republic, is one of the greatest evils." Rush to John Adams, 21 July 1789, *Letters*, 1: 523.

33. Rush to John Montgomery, 5 November 1782, *Letters*, 1: 292. See Brunhouse, *Counter-Revolution*, for a full account of the constitutional struggle in Pennsylvania. For more about Rush's role in this conflict, check the index in *Letters*.

34. Rush to Timothy Pickering, 30 August 1787; Rush to Richard Price, 2 June 1787, *Letters*, 1: 439, 418. According to L. H. Butterfield, "from 1790 onward Rush grew steadily more disillusioned about saving the world through any mundane agency. The national party warfare he witnessed during the Federalist regime seemed to him a travesty of the republican principles he had worked to establish. State politics were even more sordid, and after 1800 they grew worse rather than better" (ibid., p. lxxii).

35. Rush to Richard Price, 25 May 1786, ibid., 388.

36. Rush made this connection himself. In a letter to Noah Webster in 1789 he wrote that "having lived to see my last political wish accomplished in the change of the Constitution of Pennsylvania, I have taken leave of public life and public pursuits. Hereafter I expect to live only for the benefit of my family and my patients." 29 December 1789, ibid., p. 530.

37. Waserman, "Benjamin Rush on Government," pp. 639–40. This section of Waserman's essay is based on the lecture notes of Marcus H. Kuhl, who received an A.M. degree from the university in 1792. The notes are housed at the National Library of Medicine in Bethesda, Maryland.

38. Ibid., p. 640.

39. While Rush did not name those he thought would mislead the passions to turbulence, he sincerely believed that only those "gentlemen of the first character for virtue," who had both abilities and property were worthy of political office. See Rush to Caspar Wistar, 25 October 1785, Morris Family Papers, Quaker Collection, Haverford College Library.

40. Ibid.

41. Rush to John Adams, 12 October 1779, *Letters*, 1: 240. While nineteenth-century temperance efforts have been largely associated with religious reformers, it should be noted that Rush's concerns were political.

42. Rush to Anthony Wayne, 2 April 1777; Rush to Charles Lee, 24 October 1779, *Letters*, 1: 137, 244.

43. Rush, *Sermons to Gentlemen upon Temperance and Exercise* (Philadelphia: Printed for John Dunlap, 1772). This essay was also reprinted in London the same year under the title *Sermons to the Rich and Studious*. Rush, "Against Spirituous Liquors," *Pennsylvania Journal*, 26 June 1782. According to L. H. Butterfield, *Letters*, 1: 272, n. 1, this anonymous letter to the editor was "the first planned operation" in Rush's "long campaign against distilled spirits." Rush, *An Enquiry into the Effects of Spirituous Liquors upon the Human Body, and Their Influence upon the Happiness of Society* (Philadelphia: Thomas Bradford, n.d.). This undated tract is referred to in a letter of July 1784, though it could have been published earlier. A second edition was published in 1787, and was enlarged in 1790 and in 1791. It was also published in Edinburgh in 1791 and in 1810. Rush also had it reprinted in newspapers a number of times, including the *Pennsylvania Gazette*, 18 June 1788, where, according to Butterfield, *Letters*, 1: 521, n. 1, "it usually appeared about this season each year." A revised and enlarged version was published in 1804.

    Rush's correspondence reveals that by 1788 several religious groups, particularly the Quakers and Methodists, were taking action to prevent the sale and use of spirituous liquors. Rush to Jeremy Belknap, 6 May 1788, and 7 October 1788; Rush, "An Address Upon Subjects Interesting to Morals," 21 June 1788; Rush to John Howard, 14 October 1789, *Letters*, 1: 460, 490, 462, 527.

44. Rush, *Sermons to Gentlemen*, pp. 18–21.
45. Ibid., p. 25.
46. Rush, *An Enquiry into the Effects of Spirituous Liquors*, p. 11.
47. Rush, "An Account of the Influence of the Military and Political Events of the American Revolution upon the Human Body," *Medical Inquiries and Observations*, 2nd American ed., 3 vols. (Philadelphia: Thomas Dobson, 1794), 1: 263–78.
48. Ibid., p. 277.
49. John Hill, *The Old Man's Guide to Health and Longer Life: With Rules for Diet, Exercise, and Physic* (Philadelphia: John Dunlap, 1775). For discussions of Rush's definition of mental illness, see Eric T. Carlson and Meribeth M. Simpson, "The Definition of Mental Illness: Benjamin Rush (1745–1813)," *The American Journal of Psychiatry* 121 (1964): 209–14; and for his evolving ideas regarding the somatic treatment of mental illness, see Chris Holmes, "A Somatic Interpretation of the Psychiatry of Benjamin Rush," *American Journal of Psychiatry* 124 (1967): 133–39. After the 1793 yellow fever epidemic when Rush came to believe that "acute madness was like a state of fever, occasioned by an inflammation of the brain with an accompanying convulsion in the arterial system," he began to use the same remedies he had developed against fevers to treat mental diseases (p. 137). Rush wrote John Adams that "I have endeavored to bring them [mental diseases] down to the level of all the other diseases of the human body, and to show that the mind and body are moved by the same causes and subject to the same laws" (4 November 1812, *Letters*, 2: 1164).
50. Rush, "An Oration . . . Moral Faculty," p. 20.
51. Rush to John Adams, 13 April 1790, *Letters*, 1: 545.
52. Rush, "Information to Europeans Who Are Disposed to Migrate to the United States of America. In a Letter to a Friend in Great Britain," *Essays, Literary, Moral and Philosophical*, ed. Michael Meranze (Schenectady, N.Y.: Union College Press,

1988), pp. 118–19 (original letter written 16 April 1790). See *Letters*, 1: 557, n. 1 for the history of the circulation of this document.

53. Rush to John Adams, 15 June 1789, *Letters*, 1: 517.

54. For a sampling of works that have discussed the passionate nature of politics in the 1790s, see Marshall Smelser, "The Federalist Period as an Age of Passion," *American Quarterly* 10 (1958): 391–419; Smelser, "The Jacobin Phrenzy: Federalism and the Menace of Liberty, Equality, and Fraternity," *Review of Politics* 13 (1951): 457–82; Smelser, "The Jacobin Phrenzy: The Menace of Monarchy, Plutocracy, and Anglophilia, 1789–1798," *Review of Politics* 21 (1959): 239–58; and John R. Howe, "Republican Thought and the Political Violence of the 1790s," *American Quarterly* 19 (1967): 147–65. For an examination of how the passionate nature of politics during the 1790s contributed to a redefinition of the family and its relation to the political world, see Jan Lewis, "The Blessings of Domestic Society: Thomas Jefferson's Family and the Transformation of American Politics," in *Jeffersonian Legacies*, ed. Peter S. Onuf (Charlottesville: University Press of Virginia, 1993), pp. 109–44.

55. It seems that the street action surrounding French Ambassador Genêt's visit to Philadelphia in 1793 did scare John Adams, who wrote many years later that "the coolest and the firmest minds . . . have given their opinions to me, that nothing but the yellow fever . . . could have saved the United States from a total revolution of government." Adams to Thomas Jefferson, 30 June 1813, *The Adams-Jefferson Letters*, ed. Lester J. Cappon, 2 vols. (Chapel Hill: University of North Carolina Press, 1959), 2: 346–47.

56. Robert Lawson-Peebles, *Landscape and Written Expression* (Cambridge: Cambridge University Press, 1988), pp. 91–99.

57. It is interesting that although Lawson-Peebles recognized that Rush saw a cause and effect relationship between political disturbance and disease during the 1790s, he did not take the argument further. Instead, Lawson-Peebles argued that "yet, even with an apparently clear diagnosis of his country's ills, Rush had not been able to minister to it" (ibid., pp. 91–98; quote from p. 98).

58. Despite the fact that Rush observed in his yellow fever patients a "weak and low pulse," he came to the realization after reading Dr. Mitchell's manuscript that the resulting debility he witnessed was of the "indirect" kind, which, according to Rush, meant that the contagion "acted as a stimulus upon the whole system" (*Account*, p. 199). This debility, Rush believed, functioned as "a predisposing *cause* of illness." For a more detailed discussion of Rush's theory of disease, see Shryock, *Medicine and Society*, p. 69; and Carlson and Simpson, "Definition of Mental Illness," p. 211.

59. Rush to Julia Rush, 6 September 1793, *Old Family Letters*, p. 19.

60. Rush to John Adams, 25 November 1806, *Letters*, 2: 935.

61. Ibid., pp. 329–330.

Beyond Therapeutics: Technology and the Question of Public Health in Late-Eighteenth-Century Philadelphia

MICHAL McMAHON

UBLISHED accounts of the 1793 yellow fever epidemic document the heavy-handed and invasive approach of physicians like Benjamin Rush and the elite members of the College of Physicians. Yet the intense drama of that first and most devastating epidemic of the decade—leading not only to a war of pamphlets but also to a fictional account and a poem—have made it difficult to see beyond the physicians' ministrations. From the remarkable pamphlets published in late 1793 and 1794 to John H. Powell's vivid narrative, *Bring Out Your Dead*, published in 1949, one finds at center stage the day-to-day fight against the disease, the relative efficacy and the motivations of the different groups of caregivers, and the quarreling over competing medical approaches.[1]

Historian Charles E. Rosenberg has called for an even closer look at the early physicians' views of health and illness and the content of their well-stocked pharmacopeia and armamentaria.[2] Yet however valuable more knowledge of medical practice may be for the history of medicine, such information would add little to our understanding of the social and technical currents that stirred Philadelphia during the 1790s. From these sources came the practical responses to the series of epidemics that nearly brought the nation's largest city to its knees. Following the 1793 event, yellow fever returned with force in 1797, 1798, and 1799, decimating Philadelphia's population and leading some citizens to question the value of cities themselves.

Inflating the role of physicians obscures the effective responses made by civic officials and influential citizens to the problems of public health and urban decay that confronted Philadelphia during the decade. Nevertheless, historians of medicine have gone so far as to dismiss the role of city officials without explanation—or further investigation. Richard Shryock, a pioneer historian of medicine in the British colonies and the United States, found the "local, state, and national governments all disintegrated." Rosenberg describes "a city almost in chaos . . . administered by a completely unofficial group of public-spirited citizens." While focusing on the "great physicians," the modern chronicler of the event, John Powell, trivialized the efforts of city officials when he included them among the "little people." He placed the mayor—who, in Powell's narrative, actually emerges as a hero—in a list which includes a tavern keeper and a one-legged blacksmith.[3] When the technical story has been told, the focus has been on the Council's climactic decision in 1799 to build a centralized, steam-powered watering system. Neither the standard history of urban watering systems in the United States nor the published papers of the engineer of the waterworks discuss the eighteenth-century context and sources of that decision.[4]

These narrow approaches have had unfortunate consequences. By favoring the activities of physicians over those of city officials, we miss the opportunity to examine the roots and context of the urban crisis that gripped American cities during the late eighteenth century. By narrowing in on the waterworks built at the end of the decade, we miss the significance of the everyday activities of maintenance and upkeep which continue to form a major part of municipal engineering. Although the problems of degraded urban environments equally marked the nation's older northeastern cities of Boston and New York, it was Philadelphia's civic leaders who first launched a sustained, effective response to the question of public health. Beginning even before the fateful epidemic of 1793, the municipal government established under the charter of 1789 had begun to reorganize the city's maintenance procedures following the neglect and mismanagement of a dozen years of war and recovery. Considering the full range of responses to the yellow fever epidemics brings to the fore not only prior conditions and policy but also the critical steps taken after the 1793 epidemic to clean up the city and to construct an official apparatus for dealing with the health of the community. This broad approach also reveals how, during the years that followed, a growing awareness of the connection between wholesome water and health emerged among Philadelphia's leadership.[5]

The story of the physicians, in short, lies outside of the events that shook Philadelphia during the 1790s, and which produced the responses that would shape the nineteenth-century industrial city. For a medical story of comparable significance, one has to turn to the second half of the nineteenth century, when physicians came to accept the notion of specific disease origins and the germ theory of disease. With health rather than medicine at the center of the discussion, the historical queries raised by investigations of the yellow fever epidemics of the 1790s leads directly to both the internal improvements movement and to the struggles by city leaders and workers to ameliorate what they believed lay behind the periodic epidemics: a filthy urban environment and a dangerously polluted water supply.

THE CITY GOVERNMENT, CLEAN STREETS, AND DISEASE

Constructing a story that acknowledges the central importance of the acts of city government and the holders of public office need not deny the questionable behavior of some officials. Many members of the city council did flee the city. Governor Thomas Mifflin's flight to the countryside perhaps typified the majority response of local officials and representatives of the state government then located in Philadelphia. Mifflin hypocritically advised the city to persevere without giving so much as a coin of support. His response compared dismally to the New York City Council's gift of $5,000 to aid the nation's "seat of empire" in its moment of dire crisis. Alongside Mifflin's behavior must be placed the key roles played by members of the Council who organized to combat the 1793 epidemic, and the steps city officials took in its aftermath to refine and expand routine municipal practices for cleaning the city.

When Benjamin Rush sounded the alarm in August 1793, city officials were already struggling with the growing number of deaths resulting from the terrible disease that entered the city in late July. Rush's warning and the obvious presence of the disease led Mayor Matthew Clarkson to request advice from the College of Physicians of Philadelphia, which met on 25 August. Three days later, the Council acted on the College's report, written principally by Rush, by appointing a committee on the "malignant fever" to organize relief measures for the poor and to clean up the city. The full Council then formally adjourned, planning to hold no more official meetings until the fever abated. Just prior to adjourning, the Council affirmed by resolution the work of Clarkson, several councilmen, and the commissioners who oversaw the daily operations of the various areas of municipal concern, principally streets, water courses and drainage, solid waste removal, and security. The daily efforts of government officials to remove the dead, care for the dying, and clean the city continued into September and beyond, after the Council had formally adjourned. The mayor, with what help he could gather, began early to complement the Commissioners' work by caring for the destitute and working to improve the general state of the city.[6]

As the epidemic continued to rage, a group of councilors met on 12 September to plan a broader response from the community, one that went beyond that of the Council's Committee on Malignant Fever. The report issued by this *ad hoc* committee of the city government led to a second meeting two days later, at which a large body of citizens responded to the invitation of the mayor and Council members. Representatives came not only from Philadelphia, but also from the Northern Liberties and Southwark, the two communities on the banks of the Delaware River just above and below Philadelphia. Prominent Philadelphians who served on the Committee as private citizens ranged from merchants Stephen Girard and Thomas Wistar, to tavern owner and merchant

Israel Israel, publisher Mathew Carey, and Thomas Savery, an elderly harness maker and apothecary. Savery prescribed for the sick, operating outside the framework of the College, while his son, Benjamin, stood with Rush among that elite group of physicians. The participants at the meeting of 14 September took the name of the Council's earlier committee and established a broad, community-based Committee on Malignant Fever. In December, it once again became a Council committee, to serve until spring as the city's public health agency.[7]

Although private citizens played key roles on the committee and in battling the epidemic, members of the city government dominated its activities as they had its formation. Councilman and chemical manufacturer Samuel Wetherill chaired the initial 12 September meeting, attended also by Samuel M. Fox, head of the Bank of Pennsylvania. Fox represented a family long prominent in the city's construction trades, which had recently assumed a role in financing and governing development in the city. He remained an influential figure in the city's infrastructural development, later playing a key role in the decision to build a central water works. Wetherill, Fox, and their fellow councilors assumed prominent positions on the Committee on Malignant Fever. Mayor Clarkson chaired both the organizing meeting of 14 September and the Committee itself.[8]

Established when the summer's heat still held sway and the first frost lay several weeks ahead, the Committee took on the charge of attending "to . . . the sufferings of those afflicted with the malignant fever . . . in the city and its vicinity." In the published minutes, Committee members offered an analysis of the disease's origins and outlined the steps needed to combat its sources. Prepared in the heat of the epidemic and amid fears of foreign contagion, the Committee argued that "increased trade and population subjects the citizens to constant danger from the numbers that are daily arriving from foreign parts, where infectious disorders are frequently prevalent." The report admitted to problems on the home front when it warned against further growth, advising the community "to guard against the dangers" implicit in the increase in the size and density of the population.[9]

The notion that disease was related to cleanliness and the commitment to tightening standards grew out of discussions between the Committee on Malignant Fever and the state government during the fall of 1793. Responding to Governor Mifflin's request for advice to municipal authorities on how "to guard against a similar calamity in future," the Committee recommended that a city "health-office" be organized and given extensive responsibilities. The Committee suggested also that a "healthful spot" be found for a hospital, located outside the city, yet near enough for conveniently receiving the sick. This followed from the precedent set in late September when Mayor Clarkson and the Guardians of the Poor, a group of young men committed to public service, established a hospital at Bush Hill, a large, abandoned mansion northwest of the city.[10]

On 9 December, at its first regular meeting since the 28 August adjournment, the City Council confirmed the official nature of the Committee on Malignant Fever and adopted "measures [that would] totally . . . destroy any such infectious Matter." It directed the Committee to examine the rooms and houses where people had died of the fever and to clean out those still containing the "seeds of its infection."[11] From December through March, 1794, the City Council devised and executed ameliorative programs. As the meeting in August had confirmed the measures already taken by city officials, so did the Council's actions in March recognize the work of half a year, when it changed the name of the Committee on the Malignant Fever to the Committee of Health.[12]

Believing as they did that the epidemics were somehow related to the poor physical state of the city, Council members had already turned to the fundamental tasks of maintenance. In January 1794, they devised a long-term plan for "better cleansing the streets." A planning group of three councilors, one of whom was Samuel Fox, initially assumed responsibility. The Council directed Fox and his fellow councilors to arrange for "watering the streets by means of carts or other ways" during the summer and fall season.[13]

Within two weeks of the January meeting, the planning committee reported that the recent crisis still left the bedding and clothing of the diseased to be gathered, "smoaked and otherwise purified." The Council ordered such steps to be taken and adopted the report's more elaborate means for cleaning the city, which included dividing the city into five districts, each with a commissioner in charge. Provisions were made for five "tight carts, so as to remove the filth of the streets when in a liquid state," and five "water carts" equipped with leather buckets to water and clean the streets during the summer and fall seasons under the direction of the Mayor.[14]

Such acts were neither newly-minted with the charter issued to the city in 1789, nor with the entrance into the government during the 1790s of dynamic new men like Henry Drinker, Jr., and his brother-in-law Thomas Pym Cope, who had moved from Lancaster in 1785 to make his fortune in the region's principal city. Indeed, the city officials who responded to the crisis drew on the technical and organizational experience of many decades.[15] Water carts and leather buckets represented an approach to city problems that extended to initiatives like the legislative acts of the 1760s that gathered and refined the ordinances of a half-century into a systematic approach to such problems as waste removal, street repair and paving, and an expanding drainage network of gutters and sewers. In addition, even before the Revolution the Council had attempted to ensure the purity of the water supply by setting the depths of water wells and privy pits in the city.[16]

Ambitious public works projects had been proposed and at times carried out during the past century. Plans devised during the 1690s to convert the city's main interior cove and stream into a canal—later called the Dock—had been largely carried out. Neglect of the Dock later led to large-scale plans for rebuilding the city core, as in 1748, when a Council committee devised an engineering proposal to restore the Dock and the area around it as a multi-purpose wharving facility. In 1739, a group of citizens forced action in the Assembly in an ultimately unsuccessful attempt to remove industrial processing operations, including over half a dozen tanneries, from the heart of the city.

A project of similar scope emerged in 1791 when the projectors of a canal, seeking support from the Assembly, enhanced their chances by offering Philadelphia's city government the opportunity of drawing water from the canal to provide an external source of "wholesome water" to the city. In 1792, the Assembly chartered the company of investors and promoters of internal improvements to construct their canal along the west bank of the Schuylkill and cut east to the Delaware River across the northern boundary of the city.[17] By connecting the two rivers, the canal was to supply the city with water. Its Philadelphia-based investors perceived the canal as "a capital link in the great chain of inland navigation between our metropolis, and the Ohio and western lakes." Toward the end of the decade, the project became the first plan to be recommended by a city committee for providing pure water to the city.[18] The inability of city officials and the canal investors to agree on questions of control and ownership would in turn spur city leaders to launch the largest public works project in Philadelphia's history up to that time.

Until then, city leaders moved to reinvigorate long-established procedures for cleaning the city's streets and alleys. Although water carts were used as they had been in Europe for centuries to keep down dust created during hot, dry weather by carriages and horses, they were to be used in 1794 also to wash the streets and to carry off liquid wastes from domestic and industrial sources. The carts drew their water from public pumps that since the early 1700s had been built throughout the city. The construction and function of water wells had long been understood, as described in the edition of the *Encyclopaedia Britannica* reprinted in Philadelphia during the 1790s as "a hole underground, usually of a cylindrical figure, and walled with stone and mortar" for the purpose of collecting "the water of the strata around it." Skilled road builders, called "pavers," had immigrated into the city before mid-century, armed with techniques first honed by the Romans. Although certainly not attempting the twelve-foot depths of some Roman roads, which were made "as hard and compact as marble," pavers in eighteenth-century Philadelphia followed similar principles of first compacting the ground and then constructing a road bed with layers of rubble and stones of varying sizes bound together with mortar.[19]

The efficacy of the techniques depended directly on the degree of commitment on the part of city administrators and workers. Beginning soon after a new city government was chartered in 1789 and continuing to the end of the decade, the Councils gave evidence of a high level of commitment. This traditional approach received full expression in January 1798 when the Council once again defined the tasks of the various commissioners. Dissatisfied with the commissioners' annual accounts, the Select Council asked that detailed reports be submitted each December on the work accomplished in various areas. In seeking greater control by asking for prices for materials and the time and wages of laborers, the Council inadvertently documented the techniques used for maintaining the infrastructure of the city. The instructions for pitching and paving described the use of paving stones and gravel for streets and of bricks, lime, and sand for sewer construction; for cleaning the city, the use of flush carts and iron scrapers; for lighting and the watch, the use of oil, wicks, lamps, and watch boxes; and, for watering the city, the new wells to be dug and the bricks, pumps, and ironwork required.[20]

The Select Council's instructions revealed more than the details of traditional urban technology: they expressed the members' practical belief in the relationship of disease and health to environmental conditions. A belief that relied on a half-century of experience by city officials and physicians in dealing with the ravages of epidemic disease, the link was stated overtly only at those times when the disease struck especially hard. That yellow fever and diseases like smallpox or consumption were unrelated to personal hygiene (although smallpox was related to population density) had little to do with the efficacy of cleaning the city. Insofar as ordering the public spaces of the city did away with standing pools of water—an old complaint of city petitioners to grand juries—the Council's instructions were highly relevant to the task of combating yellow fever. In short, it is in the Philadelphia city government's responses to epidemic disease throughout the eighteenth century that is to be found its members' belief that the primary factor in the health of a community was a clean environment, and that the best means of achieving it would be through the agency of effective technique. The Englishman Edwin Chadwick expressed the matter succinctly in his famous report published in 1842:

> The great preventives, drainage, street and house cleansing by means of supplies of water and improved sewage, and especially the introduction of cheaper and more efficient modes of removing all noxious refuse from the towns, are operations for which aid must be sought from the science of the Civil Engineer, not from the physician.[21]

THE PHYSICIANS AND ENVIRONMENTAL DISEASE

In their understanding of environmental causes of disease, physicians became relevant to the crises of the 1790s. Behind the harsh treatments administered to balance the body's humors and fibrous tissues lay the belief that external conditions affected the equilibrium of the organism's functions and parts. Physicians and their patients thus tended to attribute the frequent fevers that marked the century to miasmas arising from the filth and stagnant pools scattered throughout the city. Issues of pollution naturally interested physicians, who had linked the filthy state of the habitat to repeated attacks of epidemic disease.

Men like Benjamin Franklin and Thomas Bond, Philadelphia's leading physician at mid-century, had before mid-century expressed concern over the recurring epidemics of late summer and early fall. In the early 1750s, Bond linked pollution and imbalance in the environment to imbalance in the patient, and urged a campaign to clean up the city. His concerns found powerful reinforcement during the 1762 yellow fever epidemic.[22] That experience spurred the first comprehensive efforts by the Corporation and Assembly to organize paving and cleaning of streets, removal of solid wastes, and extension of the city's drainage system. During the next few years, city officials responded to decades of controversy over the polluted stream when they converted the upper third of Dock Creek into a drainage sewer. By that time, the stream served as little more than the collective sump for Philadelphia's wastes.[23]

One of Bond's assistants during the 1762 epidemic was Benjamin Rush. Only nineteen years old at the time, Rush succeeded the older man as the leading medical personage in the city. As on most matters, Rush spoke boldly on the issue of disease origins. He rejected the idea of specific "disease entities." The "only reality" was "bodily reaction to adverse stimuli—to mental states within or to cold, miasmata, and the like without." Rush never thought of "animalcula" as a causal factor, although he had speculated that perhaps insects were related to "the dangers of marsh effluvia."[24] Although Rush did raise the question of insects in 1793, he came closer than many of his contemporaries to locating the sources of disease. Rush's beliefs that diseases came from general climatic conditions and that epidemics stemmed from effluvia or miasma rising from decaying materials may have, in strict medical terms, incorrectly explained the etiology of yellow fever. Yet belief, by physicians like Bond and Rush, in environmental sources of disease led to sound public health policy as they advocated sanitary measures to combat epidemic disease.

Richard Shryock was only partly correct when he wrote that Rush and Bond pioneered in the sanitary reform movement by advocating a clean habitat.[25] The long perspective of eighteenth-century Philadelphia reveals no sign of a reform movement, only persistent demands from citizens to the Assembly, City Corporation, and Grand Juries for cleaning up the city. Since before 1700, large numbers of citizens had periodically petitioned officials to comabt epidemic disease by removing waste or improving drainage. More accurately, then, the physicians joined their voices to those of a great number of citizens, including leading members of the merchant and artisan communities. During the 1790s, it would be physicians' ignorance of the true origins of yellow fever, combined with a recognition that disease struck hardest at poor people residing in the most polluted sections of the city, that would lend support to Council members' advocacy of measures to clean up the city.

THE QUEST FOR PURE WATER

In an era when balance pervaded public discourse, and even dictated the form of the new national government, medical analogies were often used to bolster arguments, as when one individual warned against extending "the body politic" because it would "enfeeble the circulation of its powers and energies in the extreme parts."[26] Yet city leaders had already begun to focus their efforts on specific sources of disease. Missing from the official and expert evaluations of Philadelphia's dilemma following the 1793 epidemic was the matter of the purity of the water supply. In a standard history of public health published in 1958, George Rosen acknowledged the developments in water supply made since the seventeenth century and especially in England after 1750, yet asserted that "the public health consequences of this development did not become clearly apparent until the nineteenth century."[27] Writing a half-century after Philadelphia's 1793 epidemic, Chadwick had even failed to remark on the significance of water for health—other than its use in cleaning—in his summary of the contributions of municipal engineering to public health.

Rosen's oversight could be attributed to his focus on Europe, and, in the United States, to New York City, yet it more likely stems from a common failure to acknowledge the growing awareness of the relation of wholesome water to disease after 1750. Nonetheless, the connection had been made by then. It had a number of sources, not the least of which were the opinions of medical men. Although bathing was rare among wealthy Philadelphians like Elizabeth Drinker, who took her first full bath in 1799 after a 28-year hiatus, the belief that cleanliness was critical to a healthy constitution, and that water was needed to achieve cleanliness, whether of the person or of public spaces, appeared in widely-circulated writings. To neglect cleanliness was to live in a "state of barbarity," according to William Buchan, a Scottish physician and author of the best-selling *Domestic Medicine*. When Philadelphia printer Thomas Dobson reprinted Buchan's 1769 book during the 1790s—it had first been published in Philadelphia in 1774—he reintroduced the city to an "immensely popular" book that argued the connection between pure water and health.[28]

Writers other than physicians advanced the idea, which was apparently so widely accepted as to require no elaborate arguments. References to the link between water and disease made in Philadelphia alone during the 1790s substantiate the presence of the belief. The Philadelphia poet Philip Freneau wrote during the "prevalence of a yellow fever" in 1793 of "Nature's poisons here collected / Water, earth, and air infected." A letter to *Claypoole's American Daily Advertiser* explained in 1799 that the problem lay with the poor placement of "necessaries . . . above the depth of the pumps," thereby introducing "poisons" directly "to the water, and poison is drank as well as breathed." This source had been recognized by city officials before the Revolution, of course, when they regulated the depths of wells and waste pits. There could be no more authoritative source for Philadelphians than the *Encyclopaedia Britannica*, which the printer Thomas Dobson made available during the 1790s. The lengthy entry on "Water," which chiefly discussed various methods for analyzing water and the qualities and sources of "pure water," included a substantial discussion of "putrid water." Its argument, summarized at the outset, was that "the putrescence of animal or vegetable substances" rendered water "in the highest degree pernicious to the human frame, and capable of bringing on mortal diseases even by its smell." The exhalation from polluted water was clearly secondary to its effects when ingested as a liquid. A source of its poisonous nature, the article pointed out, was the presence of animalcules, a "species of insect." Amounting to only one part in a million, the insects could make water disease-ridden even when "confined to the air."[29]

We cannot know whether anyone on the councils or the various watering committees established between 1797 and 1799 read the encyclopedia entry on water. Nor can we know whether, during the early epidemics, Council members had advanced arguments linking polluted water to disease, since Council minutes omitted the content of discussions that led to decisions. By the end of the decade, however, Council members had publicly acknowledged the link between disease and water quality. After attending chiefly to the problems of filth in the city's public spaces through most of the decade, city leaders turned to a search for pure water to prevent further epidemics.

Acknowledgement of the Councils' reasoning came first with the publication of a watering committee report in January 1798. It advised the purchase of the canal being constructed by the Delaware and Schuylkill Canal Company as the best means of securing "a sufficient quantity of wholesome water." The document demonstrated the committee's confident belief in the link between pure water and health. After iterating the need for water to clean streets, extinguish fires, and "for supplying pipes, conduits, etc. for the use of citizens," the report stated that "wholesome water . . . is now thought essential to the health of the community, and one of the means most effectual to prevent or mitigate the return of the late contagious sickness." The widespread understanding within the community of the importance of pure water was strengthened by the Committee's inclusion of a portion of a December 1797 letter received from the officers of the Canal Company in its report.[30]

Only in March 1799, after receiving a proposal from Benjamin H. Latrobe for a steam-powered waterworks to deliver Schuylkill water to the city, did the official minutes include an explicit discussion of the causes of yellow fever. In justifying their decision to build the nation's first large-scale, urban watering system—the city's most expensive public works project to date—the Select Council proclaimed the malignant fever to be "of domestic origin." Still they did not declare the connection between water and health, instead directing that workers be organized to flush the docks, common sewers, and gutters, and to sweep away the filth.[31]

In December 1799, the connection of disease to water was explicitly stated in the minutes. Following the third epidemic in as many years, the joint councils expanded the "domestic origin" argument affirmed in March to include a concrete discussion of the need for wholesome water. In a memorial to the state Assembly requesting aid in securing a water supply, the councils asserted that the loss of "many valuable Citizens" and the suspension of trade because of yellow fever required a clean water supply to prevent epidemics in the future. The councils determined this, the document declared, even as physicians continued to disagree on whether "this destructive enemy" came from without or results from "causes at home." Admitting to the diversity of opinion among other classes of citizens, the councils argued the need for "good wholesome water for drinking and culinary purposes and for the occasional flooding of the streets."[32]

Placing the need for good drinking water first in the councils' list of reasons for building a waterworks reflected not only the increasing firmness with which Philadelphia's officials accepted the link between water and disease, but directly underlay the bold decision to commit the expenditure of unheard-of sums to provide the city with wholesome water. Impelled by the devastation of the 1790s epidemics and a belief in the need for a source of pure water to prevent disease, the city moved slowly but surely toward the decision to build a watering system. Unabashedly open to the notion of governmental support for internal improvements at the city level, the councils turned no less readily to the state government. They asked the legislature for the power to promote adequate "useful improvements" and for financial assistance because, "yet tottering as our citizens are under the weight and effects of the late melancholy scene, the burthen of the work may prove too heavy for them if unaided by the fostering hand of government."[33]

Fundamental to Philadelphia's initiatives was the presence of a scientific and technological community of long standing. Familiarity with technical matters provided the means to respond to the problems of growth. The city's leadership faced an obviously unsanitary habitat and, just as obviously to these men, they possessed no reliable knowledge of the origins of disease or of dependable treatments for communicable diseases. Yet it was surely no co-incidence that the Drinker family installed the first shower on their premises in 1798 and a tub in 1803, both pioneer acts, and that their son, Henry Drinker, Jr., served with his friend, Thomas Cope, on the Councils' Watering Committee during these years.[34] These urbanites did understand technology. Men like Thomas Cope and members of old Philadelphia families like Drinker and Samuel Fox well understood the issue at hand.[35] Even when the highly-trained engineer entered the picture, Cope proved himself equal to Latrobe's hubris on the issue of engineering itself. Aware of technological means, Philadelphia's leading citizens had long been constructing their environment to sustain the urban forms that served them.[36]

For two years beginning in 1797, committees proliferated as the councils considered different sources and plans. Finally, in November 1797, the first of several joint committees was established with Samuel Fox as chair. Fox was a central figure through most of the early committee configurations and usually chaired them. The city had come a long way in the three years since Fox served on the 1794 committee that advised cleaning the streets with water carts and leather buckets. This new committee operated under Council instructions to choose a new, external source of water for the city and to build a centralized distribution system. Fox played a pivotal role during the early negotiations: he not only employed Henry Drinker, who would later be appointed to another committee under Fox, but also first brought Latrobe to Philadelphia to design a new bank building. Fox early lent his influence to the Canal Company's scheme and, in the joint committee's report of January 1798, recommended the company's plan.

The Canal Company offered to dig a small canal from their "grand reservoir"—that is, the canal linking the Schuylkill with the Delaware. The branch canal would be "cut from north to south, along Broad Street, the whole breadth of the city, and bridged over at the crossing of each street." Water discharged at a rate of a half a million cubic feet per hour would at first be used to wash the streets and extinguish fires and later would be distributed by means of "pipes and conduits and fountains." The committee apparently found the plan unobjectionable, yet its recommendation that all of the shares of the Canal Company be purchased met opposition from the company's investors, delaying a decision.[37]

In the month of the Committee's recommendation, the Councils were receiving citizens' petitions asking for a water supply by "canals or otherways."

Although the Company soon agreed that the City could purchase the entire stock owned by investors, by the next fall, the Councils asked a committee of Drinker, Fox, Cope, and others to use a nearby spring, Spring Mill to the north, to supply the city with water. Other proposals began to surface. Joseph Huntley of Connecticut offered a scheme based on using the Schuylkill by means of "an improvement on the mode of raising water from rivers to a height above its level."[38]

Nothing won over the Councils until January 1799, when a committee charged with locating a "competent person" submitted to the Councils a communication received from Latrobe, "a gentleman of scientific eminence." Latrobe's observations appeared to the committee to be "highly useful, important and interesting." Reacting as they had not done before, the Councils resolved to publish Latrobe's communication, a pamphlet-length essay entitled *View of the Practicability and Means of Supplying the City of Philadelphia with Wholesome Water.*[39] Once committed to Latrobe's plan, the joint committee urged that no more delays occur in raising money through a public subscription.

Latrobe presented his solution as "the only means." His plan proposed a steam-powered system which would draw water from the Schuylkill into a settling basin at the foot of Chestnut Street to allow for sedimentation, then force it by aqueduct to a point in the center of the town where a second steam engine would pump the water into a raised reservoir. Since filtration systems were only then being introduced into England—the first filtered system of a size to supply an entire town was completed at Paisley, Scotland, in 1804—Latrobe understandably did not discuss the idea. In any case, the purity of the Schuylkill's water required no filtering.[40] Although he would use the same source as Huntley had proposed, Latrobe chose steam power over water power and aggressively pressed his choice to the Councils, arguing that "to do this in sufficient quantity, very powerful machinery will be required; and, I am very certain, that human ingenuity has not hitherto invented any thing capable of producing the proposed effect with constancy, certainty, and adequate force, excepting the steam-engine." In all species of machinery in which "mechanical powers alone operate," as in a water-powered system, the size of the works increased in proportion to the power required. Yet "in the chemical operation of the steam-engine, power is increased in a ration far outstripping the bulk and the price of the engine." Latrobe's optimism was unbounded, for he promised also that "when the first expense is incurred, the two men that are necessary to tend the smallest can manage the most gigantic mechanism."[41]

Besides arguing for the greater efficiency of steam power in its manpower requirements, consistency, and economy, Latrobe attacked the underpinning of technologies that relied on the "vagaries of nature," such as the "variable seasons" or the "natural advantages of the site." These sentiments reveal much about the engineering judgments Latrobe brought to his design, which

109

he offered along with a detailed attack on water power, because the idea of erecting "water-works to be driven by one of the two rivers" had been promoted as "worthy of consideration."

To aid the Councils in their deliberations and to bolster his argument for steam engines, Latrobe provided in March *An Answer to the Joint Committee* on the subject of "a plan for supplying the city with water," to which he appended "An Account of Steam Engines, etc." In the Account, Latrobe listed six areas of the cities of London and Westminster which were "in part supplied with water" by steam engines. It was a compelling list, reiterating all the components of Latrobe's proposed system: raised reservoirs, cast iron mains, wooden pipes. His final example was preceded by the comment that "every one who has been at Paris" has heard the cries of the waterporters, "whose cry had something remarkable in it, to the ear of a foreigner." Yet because of their inconvenience, an "extraordinary" steam engine was erected for raising and distributing water by pipes to the city. He concludes with a final, disingenuous comment that

> Soon after the invention, steam engines were justly considered as dangerous, man had not yet learned to control the immense power of steam, and now and then they did a little mischief. A steam engine is, at present, as tame and innocent as a clock.[42]

If the engineer's proposal did not seem disingenuous to the councilors at the time, it soon would as problems abounded. Wooden pipes left to dry in the open air burst as water entered them when laid underground; the raised reservoir at Centre Square soon proved inadequate to the needs of the city; and the vaunted steam engines fell far short of the efficency and reliability of even the wooden clockworks of the time. As to their tameness, excessive fuel consumption, breakdowns, and accidents tried, and sometimes killed, the workers charged with their operation and maintenance.[43] In fact, it was not until the 1820s, when the pumping station was moved upriver and converted to water power, and steam engines assumed a supplemental role, that the Philadelphia Waterworks operated in the black.

The path the Councils followed to a solution in the crisis can be seen now as smooth and consistent. When they confronted a confusion of choices and advocates, city leaders determined to consult an expert. Latrobe's arguments for the efficiency in terms of both cost and effectiveness of steam engines seemed as sound to the councilors as to the young British engineer. Yet Latrobe's several assurances about costs seemed not to matter to the Councils, which apparently believed that loans, taxes, subscriptions, and dedicated fees would be ample. Indeed, the habitual raising of estimated costs, while disturbing, won continued acceptance from Philadelphia's leaders. When the Federalist councilors lost control of the city government in the 1801 elections

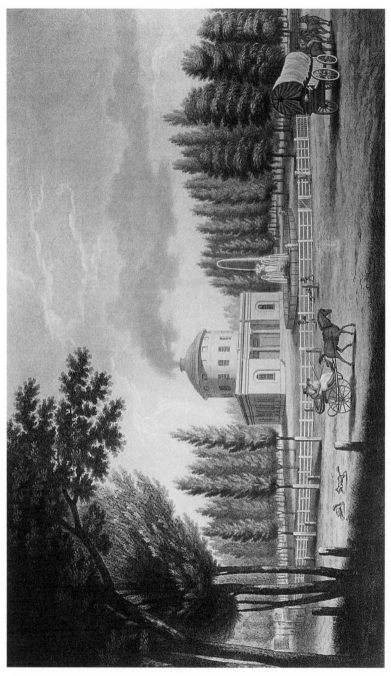

View of the Water Works of Centre Square, by C. Trebout after J.J. Barralet. Courtesy of the Library Company of Philadelphia.

to the Democratic opposition, Latrobe found even greater support. His first estimate had amounted to $127,000 and the Councils had granted $150,000. In 1798, the first Joint Committee headed by Fox had recommended the Canal Company's plan at an estimated cost of $350,000, which the Committee found acceptable. Even the final cost reported in 1801 of $220,000 seemed not to disturb the Councils. Cope, who wrote in his diary throughout 1800 about the need for money, seemed most angered by Latrobe's personal bearing: he found the engineer to be "a cunning, witful, dissimulating fellow, possessing more ingenuity than honesty."[44]

Latrobe's reasoning revealed a deeper, more timeless conflict than the arguments over engineering designs and costs for centralized water supply systems. Behind the crisis of the city in 1800 lay the old conflict between the city and nature, and between private gain and public purposes. Philadelphia still hugged the banks of the Delaware, crowding its 68,000 inhabitants into less than half of the town plan laid out by William Penn and his company. Because the city continued to grow in area as well as density, it had long since strained the limits of the aquifer on which the city had for so long relied. For an equally long time, Philadelphia's leaders had been mechanically altering its natural site with the construction of subterranean drainage networks and a system of streets and gutters, and by prescribing depths for wells and privy pits. In the matter of water, scarcity and pollution had been realities since mid-century. By the end of the 1700s, following a century of struggling over the source of the nearly annual visitations of malignant fever, water had joined filthy streets in the minds of the city's leaders as the chief culprit in a crisis that gripped the nation's largest city.

The cumulative impact of endemic and epidemic disease was felt more acutely during the last decade of the eighteenth century than at any previous time in the city's history. As had happened several times since the city was founded in 1682, the physical habitat had simply collapsed before a pattern of growth that constantly wracked the city with new levels of congestion. Simply put, social, economic, and institutional arrangements allowed and encouraged a degree of residential and industrial density that the land could not support. The same arrangements conspired to minimize funding for the mundane work of maintenance and upkeep and, in the late 1790s, to lavish funds on an unprecedentedly large-scale, steam-powered system which was untried in the experience of the entire country, and only recently tried in the Old World.

The terrible yellow fever attack of 1793 defined the last decade of the century: still fresh in the memory of the inhabitants in 1800, it added force to their responses to the milder epidemics that returned in succeeding years, giving support to bold urban initiatives, and winning acceptance from a city whose industrial interests had earlier thwarted similar projects. Working to improve maintenance and re-establish traditional technical practices after a dozen years of haphazard administration, the councilmen knew the real problem had never been the epidemics, however terrible their toll on the city's population and fortunes.

After the epidemics of 1797 and 1798, Council members acted as if the problem was systemic, not specific to "animacula," or even to a pile of coffee rotting on a wharf, as Rush had feared in 1793. Besides, mosquitoes bred in standing pools of water in a habitat in which flooded basements were tolerated in the packed tenements and breweries and warehouses of Water Street, where the sickness hit hardest. The physicians, city officials, and nurses and helpers who entered the streets and houses of the dead and dying experienced at first hand the results of dense settlement patterns. General concerns about the future of cities in the face of increased population and density had been expressed by Benjamin Franklin as early as the 1750s, when he feared for the future of the country in the face of an expanding population.[45]

Others crossed the gap from experience to thought, raising concerns about the viability of cities themselves, beside which the medical and engineering solutions paled, and revealing a moment in which the very progress and change so ardently sought became fearful. In 1793, the Committee on Malignant Fever feared growth in the form of recent immigrants coming to the city from foreign ports, especially from Santo Domingo. The Committee warned the governor about the "increasing trade of the city, and the great number of people who are daily arriving," and in a report to the Council in December located the source of the disease in the very nature of urban settlement, citing the crowding found in "all great commercial cities."[46] One citizen, Ebenezer Hazard, took the extreme position that the experience of 1793 ought to inhibit the "prevailing taste for enlarging Philadelphia, and crowding so many human beings together on so small a part of the earth." He recommended that Americans reject the "fashions of the Old World in building great cities."[47]

Patterns of growth in eighteenth-century Philadelphia, which were determined largely by the private sector, reflected an approach to municipal development that since the late 1600s had become the warp and woof of British American society. The patterns reveal a transformation in which social and environmental aspects of everyday life were subordinated to the interests of private purposes. In Pennsylvania, the seeds had come with the ideological and cultural baggage brought by settlers since the late 1600s. Early expressions of capitalism and possessive individualism had sprouted through the 1700s as both ideas and behaviors. They would flourish during the decades following the Revolution as legal judgments, rendered across the expanding frontier of the United States, encoded the triumph of privatism in public life.[48]

Philadelphia's health crises in the 1790s recommend an exploration of the social, organizational, and technical bases of the urban order. These will be found, moreover, in the everyday activities of maintenance and upkeep as much as in large-scale engineering works. Gender perhaps plays a role here, linking concepts of public health to the notion of "municipal housekeeping," which was introduced a century later when urban conditions became a key concern of social reformers. The phrase carries explanatory power since, at either end of the century, a housekeeping metaphor would find scant acceptance in a social and economic order defined mostly by capitalism and large-scale internal improvements projects. The pioneer attempt at canal building and the construction of a centralized watering system in late eighteenth-century Philadelphia appear as clear harbingers of the future. At the same time, insofar as urban housekeeping chores would assume a place in a social and physical world dominated by private economic development, the events of the 1790s projected them as the tasks of a subordinate and often neglected servant.

NOTES

1. Besides John H. Powell, *Bring Out Your Dead: The Great Plague of Yellow Fever in Philadelphia in 1793* (Philadelphia: University of Pennsylvania Press, 1949); see *Minutes of the Proceedings of the Committee . . . on the Malignant Fever* (Philadelphia: City of Philadelphia, 1848), hereafter *Committee on Malignant Fever;* Mathew Carey, *A Short Account of the Malignant Fever, Lately Prevalent in Philadelphia, in the Year 1793* (Philadelphia: Mathew Carey, 1794); and Richard Allen and Absalom Jones, *A Narrative of the Proceedings of the Black People during the Late Awful Calamity in Philadelphia in the Year 1793* (1794; reprint, Philadelphia: Independence National Historical Park, 1993). Charles Brockden Brown's novel, *Arthur Mervyn; Or Memoirs of the Year 1793*, 2 vols. (Port Washington, N.Y.: Kennikat Press, 1963), first published in 1799 and 1800, and Philip Freneau's poem, "Pestilence," written during the epidemic and reprinted in Powell, p. xxvi, strike more closely at the real issues raised by the crisis.

2. Charles E. Rosenberg, "The Therapeutic Revolution: Medicine, Meaning, and Social Change in Nineteenth-Century America," in Rosenberg, *Explaining Epidemics and Other Studies in the History of Medicine* (Cambridge: Cambridge University Press, 1992), pp. 9–31. By 1850, Rosenberg explains, a "therapeutic revolution" based on the idea of specific disease entities had begun to lead physicians away from the invasive therapies recommended by holistic theories—and from the theories as well.

3. Powell, *Bring Out Your Dead*, p. vii; Richard H. Shryock, *Medicine and Society in America: 1660–1860* (New York: New York University Press, 1960), pp. 94–95; Charles E. Rosenberg, *The Cholera Years: The United States in 1832, 1849 and 1866* (Chicago: University of Chicago Press, 1962), p. 82.

4. Nelson Manfred Blake, *Water for the Cities: A History of the Urban Water Supply Problem in the United States* (Syracuse, NY: Syracuse University Press, 1956); *The Engineering Drawings of Benjamin Henry Latrobe*, edited with an introductory essay by Darwin H. Stapleton (New Haven: Yale University Press, 1980). For more on the 1790s context, see A. Michal McMahon's " 'Small Matters': Benjamin Franklin, Philadelphia,

and the Progress of Cities," *Pennsylvania Magazine of History and Biography* 116 (1992): 157–182, and " 'Publick Service' versus 'Mans Property': Dock Creek and the Origins of Urban Technology in 18th-Century Philadelphia," in *Early American Technology: Making and Doing Things from the Colonial Era to 1850*, ed. Judith McGaw (Chapel Hill: University of North Carolina Press, 1994).

5. New York's government similarly responded to yellow fever in the 1790s by creating committees of health which had evolved into quasi-independent Boards of Health by the 1830s. See Rosenberg, *The Cholera Years*. See also George Rosen, *A History of Public Health* (1958; reprint, Baltimore: Johns Hopkins University Press, 1993).

6. Minutes, Philadelphia Common Council, 28 August 1793, Philadelphia City Archives, hereafter PCA. The Common Council was Philadelphia's only council until 1796, when a Select Council was created to replace the Aldermen. For the work of the mayor and others, see Powell, *Bring Out Your Dead*, passim.

7. Minutes, Philadelphia Common Council, 28 August 1793, PCA.

8. *Committee on Malignant Fever*, 14 September 1793, p. 110.

9. Ibid. For an account of the debate over origins, see Martin S. Pernick, "Politics, Parties, and Pestilence: Yellow Fever in Philadelphia and the Rise of the First Party System," *William and Mary Quarterly* 29 (1972): 559–586, and reprinted in this volume.

10. Powell, *Bring Out Your Dead*, p. 8 ff.; *Committee on Malignant Fever*, 19 November 1793, pp. 135, 140.

11. Minutes, Common Council, 9 December 1793, PCA.

12. Ibid., 24 March 1794, PCA.

13. Ibid., 6 January 1794, PCA. Alderman George Roberts and Robert Waln served with Fox.

14. Ibid., 20 January 1794, PCA.

15. Ignoring or misinterpreting the responses of the political and governmental officials to the epidemics of the 1790s has been typical. Blake (*Water for the Cities*, pp. 3–17) links the 1799 waterworks decision to the 1790s epidemics, yet discusses the 1793 epidemic only from the perspective of the contemporary pamphlets and the medical views of the physicians, introducing no other parties or responses until turning to the Council's initiative at the end of the decade. Although he mentions several technical measures taken by the Council prior to the waterworks decision in discussing the technical antecedents to the 1799 act, he points to European precedents and to the attempt to build a steam-powered water supply system for New York City before the Revolution (pp. 9, 17). In the chapter relating the story of the Philadelphia works, moreover, he emphasizes "the ingenuity of Benjamin Latrobe" rather than the commitments of city leaders who hired him.

16. See McMahon, " 'Publick Service' versus 'Man's Property,' " and Charles S. Olton, "Philadelphia's First Environmental Crisis," *Pennsylvania Magazine of History and Biography* 98 (1974): 90–100.

17. Journal, Pennsylvania House of Representatives, 17, 19, 21, 22 December 1791, 20 January 1792, 2, 10 April 1792.

18. William Smith, Chairman of Delaware and Schuylkill Canal Navigation to the Councils of the City of Philadelphia, 19 December 1797, in *Report of the Joint Com-*

mittee of the Select and Common Councils on the Subject of Bringing Water to the City (Philadelphia: n.p., 1798), p. 8.

19. *Encyclopaedia; or, a Dictionary of Arts, Sciences and Miscellaneous Literature* (Philadelphia: Thomas Dobson, 1791–1797), vols. 16, "Roads," and 18, "Water Wells."

20. Minutes, Select Council, 9 January 1798, PCA. In April 1796, the Assembly amended the 1789 charter to, among other matters, establish a twelve-person Select Council, to be elected on the same day as the members of the Common Council and to possess the same qualifications as state senators; see J. Lowber, ed., *Ordinances of the Corporation of and Acts of the Assembly Relating to the City of Philadelphia* (Philadelphia: n.p., 1812), pp. 89–90.

21. Quoted in Rosen, *History of Public Health*, p. 191; see also Ivan Illich, *Limits to Medicine: Medical Nemesis, the Expropriation of Health* (London: Boyers, 1976), p. 7. Illich cites a number of modern studies from different countries to support the assertion that "the environment [is the] primary determinant of the state of general health of any population."

22. For details of physicians' responses to this event, see Carl Bridenbaugh, *Rebels and Gentlemen: Philadelphia in the Age of Franklin* (New York: Reynal and Hitchcock, 1942), p. 295, and chapter 11. Bridenbaugh cites Bond's "Essay on the Utility of Clinical Lectures," delivered in Philadelphia on 6 November 1766. See also Roslyn Stone Wolman, "Some Aspects of Community Health in Colonial Philadelphia" (Ph.D. diss., University of Pennsylvania, 1974).

23. For a modern account of the Dock, see McMahon, " 'Publick Service' versus 'Mans Property.' "

24. Rush quoted in Shryock, *Medicine and Society*, p. 71.

25. Ibid., p. 102.

26. Quoted in Robert H. Wiebe, *The Opening of American Society: From the Adoption of the Constitution to the Eve of Disunion* (New York: Alfred A. Knopf, 1984), p. 9.

27. Rosen, *History of Public Health*, p. 101.

28. William Buchan, *Domestic Medicine; Or, the Family's Physician: Being an Attempt to Render the Medical Art More Generally Useful* (Edinburgh: Balfour, Auld, and Smellie, 1769); the characterization is from Richard L. and Claudia L. Bushman, "The Early History of Cleanliness in America," *Journal of American History* 74 (1988): 1223.

29. Freneau quoted in Powell, *Bring Out Your Dead*, p. xxvi; *Claypoole's American Daily Advertiser*, 8 January 1799, quoted in Blake, *Water for the Cities*, p. 11; *Encyclopaedia*, vol. 18, "Water."

30. *Report of the Joint Committee of the Select and Common Councils on the Subject of Bringing Water to the City* (Philadelphia: n.p., 1798), pp. 3–5.

31. Minutes, Select Council, 2 March 1799. Latrobe's proposal, dated 2 March, is entitled *An Answer to the Joint Committee of the Select and Common Councils of Philadelphia on the Subject of a Plan for Supplying the City with Water, etc.* (Philadelphia: n.p., 1799).

32. Minutes, Select Council, 5 December 1799, PCA.

33. Ibid.

34. Bushman and Bushman, "Early History of Cleanliness," pp. 1214–1215.

35. Gideon Sjoberg, *The Pre-Industrial City: Past and Present* (Glencoe, Ill.: Free Press, 1960), p. 95, describes the individuals facing these conditions in ignorance of

medical causes and treatment methods "preindustrial urbanites." The Philadelphians' very familiarity with the technical aspects of urban systems and their acceptance of an environmental explanation for disease marked them, instead, as industrial urbanites.

36. See Elizabeth Gray Kogan Spera, "Building for Business: The Impact of Commerce on the City Plan and Architecture of the City of Philadelphia" (Ph.D. diss., University of Pennsylvania, 1980). See also Thomas Cope's detailed, critical report on Nicholas Roosevelt's Soho (steam engine) Works in New Jersey, 1801, PCA.

37. *Report of the Joint Committee . . . on the Subject of Bringing Water to the City*, p. 9.

38. Minutes, Select Council, 9, 18, 31 January 1798, 15 February 1798, 28 November 1798, and 18 December 1798.

39. Minutes, Select Council, 3 January 1799, PCA.

40. Moses Nelson Baker, *The Quest for Pure Water: The History of Water Purification From the Earliest Records to the Twentieth Century* (New York: American Water Works Association, 1948), p. 64.

41. Benjamin Henry Latrobe, *View of the Practicability and Means of Supplying the City of Philadelphia with Wholesome Water* (Philadelphia: Printed by Zachariah Poulson, Jr., 1799), pp. 5, 8.

42. Ibid., 14; Latrobe, *An Answer to the Joint Committee of the Select and Common Councils of Philadelphia*, pp. 5–7.

43. Blake, *Water for the Cities*, pp. 36–40. For an account of the two men who suffocated while cleaning a boiler, see *Philadelphia Merchant: The Diary of Thomas P. Cope, 1800–1851*, ed. Eliza Cope Harrison (South Bend, Indiana: Gateway Editions, 1978), p. 51.

44. *Report of the Committee for the Introduction of Wholesome Water into the City of Philadelphia* (Philadelphia: n.p., 1801). For the Canal Company estimate, see *Report of the Joint Committee . . . on the Subject of Bringing Water to the City*, p. 7; *Philadelphia Merchant*, p. 57.

45. See McMahon, " 'Small Matters.' "

46. *Committee on Malignant Fever*, 19 November 1793, pp. 140, 199.

47. Quoted in Powell, *Bring Out Your Dead*, p. 276.

48. For the situation in late eighteenth-century Philadelphia, see Kogan Spera, "Building for Business." Morton J. Horwitz, *The Transformation of American Law, 1780–1860* (Cambridge: Harvard University Press, 1977), locates the movement away from the distributive role of English common law to the privileging of economic development, to changes in judicial judgements beginning in the late eighteenth century. For the long history behind this transformation, see Christopher Hill, *The Century of Revolution, 1603–1714* (Edinburgh: T. Nelson, 1961) and *The World Turned Upside Down: Radical Ideas During the English Revolution* (New York: Viking Press, 1972). For early Pennsylvania, see Gary B. Nash, *Quakers and Politics: Pennsylvania, 1681–1726* (Princeton: Princeton University Press, 1968), and Frederick Tolles, *Meeting House and Counting House: The Quaker Merchants of Colonial Philadelphia, 1682–1763* (Chapel Hill: University of North Carolina Press, 1948). For a specific case, see McMahon, " 'Publick Service' Versus 'Mans Property,' " on the political struggle between wealthy tanners and the residents and artisans of central Philadelphia in 1739.

Politics, Parties, and Pestilence: Epidemic Yellow Fever in Philadelphia and the Rise of the First Party System*

MARTIN S. PERNICK**

HE omens were not auspicious for Philadelphia in the summer of 1793. Unusually large flocks of migrating pigeons filled the daytime sky. By night a comet streaked the heavens. Increased numbers of cats were dying, their bodies putrefying in the streets and sinkholes, as the rains that usually washed them away were replaced by prolonged drought. Most ominously, the swarms of flies seemingly indigenous to the city had been driven off by a dense mass of "moschetoes" that hung over the city like a cloud.[1] Warned by these signs and portents, the learned Philadelphia medical community had prepared itself for the appearance of a somewhat more virulent strain of "autumnal fever" than was usual. By early August, though, the doctors were puzzling over isolated cases of a new disease involving yellowing of the skin and vomiting of an unknown black substance. On 19 August, Dr. Benjamin Rush, signer of the Declaration of Independence and dean of Philadelphia medicine, proclaimed that yellow fever had returned to the city for the first time since 1762.

Initial disbelief turned rapidly to panic as the death toll mounted. By the end of the month between 140 and 325 Philadelphians had died of the fever. On one October day, 119 dead were buried. Between 19 August and 15 November, 10 to 15 percent of the estimated 45,000 Philadelphians perished, while another 20,000, including most government officials, simply fled.[2] An extralegal committee of citizen volunteers, called upon by the mayor following the hasty departure of the regular municipal officers, gradually brought the panic under control. Growing slowly from a nucleus of ten men who an-

*Revised by the author and reprinted with permission from the *William and Mary Quarterly*, 3rd ser., 29 (1972): 559–586.

**I would like to thank Eric L. McKitrick for his guidance and encouragement at every stage of this project.

swered Mayor Matthew Clarkson's 10 September call, the committee commandeered the vacant Bush Hill estate for use as a hospital, set up an orphanage, distributed food, firewood, clothes, and medicine to the poor, buried the abandoned corpses, and undertook a complete cleanup of the city.[3]

Good intentions and hard work were not enough; the hospital could do little when no cure was known. Sanitary efforts were random at best when no one understood the cause of the sickness. The city of Philadelphia needed immediate resolution of three crucial medical questions: what caused the fever and how might its spread and recurrence be averted? how should the sick be treated? and should the people evacuate or stay?

Philadelphia was the medical capital of the United States. Franklin's Pennsylvania Hospital, the prestigious College of Physicians, and the American Philosophical Society combined to attract to the city the best of the new nation's scientific and medical talent. But the medical problems posed by yellow fever were simply not solvable by even the best eighteenth-century physicians—or, more accurately, medical science alone provided no definitive way of choosing from among the scores of conflicting causes, preventives, and cures, each presented as gospel by its learned advocates. This uncertainty provided the opening by which influences initially quite removed from medical science entered the medical debate.[4]

The yellow fever epidemic of 1793 provides an early example of the complex links between health and politics in American society. In addition, the epidemic reveals the respective roles of local and national events in the creation of America's first two-party system. Philadelphia in 1793 was not only the medical center of America but the political capital of a new republic as well. And in politics as in medicine, the presence of a large body of experts did little to expedite agreement. In fact, 1793 found the political leadership of the nation more divided than at any time in its short past. The year began amid an increasingly bitter verbal duel between Treasury Secretary Alexander Hamilton, writing in John Fenno's *Gazette of the United States*, and Secretary of State Thomas Jefferson, whose views appeared in Philip Freneau's *National Gazette*. The battle, begun over fiscal policy, took on added significance with the news at mid-spring that Revolutionary France had executed America's benefactor, Louis XVI, and had declared war on England. Jefferson and his followers feared English "monarchism" as much as Hamilton and his supporters detested French "anarchy." The arrival of Citizen Genêt, the new French Republican Minister to the United States, inspired sympathetic popular demonstrations in Philadelphia and elsewhere, events organized in part by the newly formed Pennsylvania Democratic Society. The exact purposes of this organization may well have been as unclear to the founders as they are to modern historians, but everyone agreed that it was pro-French and pro-Republican.[5]

In spite of such signs of pro-French sympathy, Jefferson's political standing underwent a marked decline in the summer of 1793. Hamilton gained increased influence over foreign policy within the administration following the April Neutrality Proclamation, while Genêt's rapid success in alienating almost everyone in America further discouraged Jefferson. On 31 July, Jefferson notified Washington of his intention to resign by year's end.

Local Philadelphia politics grew more involved following the arrival in early August of over two thousand French refugees from the black revolution in Haiti. Unlike the earlier royalist refugees, the new arrivals included many white radicals and moderates, ousted when the slaves seized control of the revolutionary movement.[6]

Both Hamilton and Jefferson feared dividing the young Republic, but their debate provided the core around which local and congressional factions crystalized to form the first institutional American party system. As Jeffersonians became Democratic-Republicans and Hamiltonians became Federalists, both sought to arouse public interest by taking sides in a variety of local or nonpolitical disputes. Local factions likewise often tried to identify their cause with a national party for ideological, rhetorical, political, or moral support against their local rivals. In either case local antagonisms were deepened and prolonged while the national party gained new grassroots significance.[7] Not surprisingly, the national parties first found themselves embroiled in local issues in the capital city of Philadelphia. The medical controversies generated by the 1793 epidemic over the cause of the disease, its proper treatment, and the conduct of those caught in the crisis, thereby became an integral chapter in the history of the first party system.

DIRTY STREETS OR DIRTY FOREIGNERS?: THE CAUSE

Since it was not until 1901 that Walter Reed demonstrated the process by which the *Aëdes aegypti* mosquito transmits yellow fever from an infected person to a healthy one, Philadelphia physicians of 1793 divided bitterly over the cause of the epidemic. Doctors who saw the roots of the disease in domestic causes—the poor sanitation, unhealthy location, or climatic conditions of Philadelphia itself—disputed those who placed the blame on the unhealthy state of the still disembarking refugees and their ships. In fact, both sides were right, since a yellow fever epidemic requires both locally bred mosquitoes and an initial pool of infected persons, such as the exiled Haitians. In 1793, however, there was simply no known medical theory to resolve the dispute.[8] The etiological debate revealed, moreover, a medical community split along partisan political lines. In general, Republican physicians, including the refugee doctors, believed the fever to be local. The "importationists" were almost all nonpartisans or Federalists.

Dr. Michael Leib, a founder of all three branches of the Philadelphia Democratic Society and a member of the key correspondence committee of the "mother society," argued the domestic origin case before the College of Physicians. Joining him was his old professor, Dr. Rush, an outspoken opponent of Hamilton. Rush, a founding fellow of the College, leader of the medical school faculty, and probably the best known physician in Philadelphia, insisted that "miasmata" from local swamps and "effluvia" from unsanitary docks bred the fever. A second member of the Democrats' correspondence committee, Dr. James Hutchinson, who as Secretary of the College and Physician of the Port was responsible for deciding to admit or bar the refugee ships, reported to Pennsylvania Governor Thomas Mifflin on 26 August, "It does not seem to be an imported disease; for I have learned of no foreigners or sailors that have hitherto been infected." Dr. Jean Devèze, himself a refugee, attributed importationism to ignorance and party influence.[9]

The advocates of importation included Philadelphia's lone confessed Federalist physician, Dr. Edward Stevens, a future diplomat and close boyhood friend of Hamilton. The other leading importationists were Drs. Adam Kuhn, Isaac Cathrall, and William Currie. Although prominent in the profession, they took no part in party politics in 1793. On 26 November, after Hutchinson's death in the epidemic enabled Kuhn and his supporters to gain a majority, the College of Physicians passed a resolution firmly asserting, "No instance has ever occurred of the disease called the *yellow fever*, having been generated in this city, or in any other parts of the United States . . . but there have been frequent instances of its having been imported." The resolution was the work of Drs. Thomas Parke, John Carson, and Samuel P. Griffitts, none of whom was politically active in 1793.[10] Benjamin Rush had resigned from the College a few days earlier. Benjamin Smith Barton was the only Republican physician in Philadelphia to support importation in this epidemic.[11] (See Table 1.)

Politics entered the issue by different doors with different doctors. As a topic for medical debate "The Origin of Pestilential Fevers" was an old favorite, and several physicians were committed to one side or the other before 1793. One such was Benjamin Rush. His 1789 comments belittling both importationism and its advocates created hostilities which may help explain why few importationists would join Rush in the Jeffersonian councils.[12]

For most physicians, though, the whole issue remained a somewhat remote subject for scholarly speculation until the crisis of 1793 suddenly forced each practitioner to choose a course of immediate action. Many turned for guidance to trusted colleagues—teachers and friends whose opinions on medical, political, and other matters they had shared in the past.[13] In addition, Republican doctors were the most likely to have come in contact with the localist doctrines which dominated French medicine. In the case of Dr. Hutchinson, politics may have influenced medical decisions more directly. An

TABLE 1. 1793 Party Affiliations of Physicians Who Expressed an Opinion on the Cause of Yellow Fever

	Republicans	*Federalists*	*Uncommitted*
Importationists—10	1	1	8
Domestic Origin—14	6	0	8

Note: Twenty-four Philadelphia physicians, the most prominent third of the practicing healers in town, left evidence of their opinions on the cause of the fever. One-third of this medical elite was actively involved in the earliest stages of party building. The prominence of this elite gave their views social significance despite their lack of statistical significance.

importationist prior to the epidemic, the Republican port physician apparently switched to localism to avoid closing the city to the French refugees.[14]

Like the physicians, the political leaders of Philadelphia split by party over the cause of the fever. Although Republican editor Freneau vehemently condemned the disputes of the medical men, declaring that "no circumstance has added more to the present calamity," he actually strongly supported a local origin. He made his viewpoint clear in the following poem:

Doctors raving and disputing,
Death's pale army still recruiting—
    What a pother
    One with t'other!
Some a-writing, some a-shooting.

Nature's poisons here collected,
Water, earth, and air infected—
    O, what a pity
    Such a City,
Was in such a place erected![15]

On 23 September, the *National Gazette* published a discussion of more than a dozen theories of the origin of the disease without once mentioning the possibility of its being imported.[16] In medicine as in politics only one's opposition was seen as the "divisive faction." Local Republican civic leaders like editor Andrew Brown and merchants John Swanwick and Stephen Girard supported Dr. Devèze's explanation that burying the dead inside the city had produced the disease. Jefferson explained to Madison that the fever was "generated in the filth of Water Street."[17]

On the other hand, Philadelphia Federalists John Fenno, Oliver Wolcott, Thomas Willing, Benjamin Chew, Levi Hollingsworth, J. B. Bordley, Ebenezer

Hazard, Bishop William White, and printer Benjamin Johnson led their party in publicly proclaiming yellow fever a foreign disease.[18] In his days as a Federalist after 1794, William "Peter Porcupine" Cobbett, the Anglo-American pamphleteer, penned a series of libelous attacks on Rush's theories. But in 1793, as a supplicant of the patronage of Secretary Jefferson and a tutor to the refugees, Cobbett spoke of the yellow fever as a typical product of the unhealthy American climate.[19]

More than one-third of the most prominent national and local political leaders in Philadelphia took a public position on the cause of the epidemic. With few exceptions the Republicans backed a domestic source of the fever, while Federalists largely blamed importation. Governor Mifflin, who endorsed importation theories, has been called a Republican although he usually appeared as the non-partisan "Father of his State." Benjamin Franklin Bache, editor of the Republican *General Advertiser*, believed the disease imported but blamed the *British* West Indies, later calling the fever "a present from the English." The least typical was Republican printer Mathew Carey, who included his native Ireland as well as the French islands among the possible sources of the fever.[20] Timothy Pickering, an intimate friend of Dr. Rush, was probably the only Federalist leader in Philadelphia to claim the yellow fever as a domestic disease.[21]

The party leaders, moreover, moved rapidly to exploit the many political implications they discovered in the medical controversy. Federalists used the importation doctrine to back demands for the quarantine or exclusion of the radical French, and for limitations on trade with the French islands, while Republican merchants saw importationism as a cover for plans to wreck their lucrative trade with the West Indies. Girard and Dr. Devèze denounced the proposed quarantine as "disastrous to commerce." In June 1798, during the "Quasi-War" with France, the newly drafted quarantine laws were in fact successfully invoked to block the immigration of suspected Haitian subversives.[22]

A novel twist was provided by Dr. Currie's theory that the disease originated on board the French privateer *Sans Culotte*, which brought a prize to Philadelphia in July. Accusing both the French and Port Physician Hutchinson, the Federalists charged that sickness on the ship had been covered up to protect the Republican political and financial stake in her activities. Benjamin Johnson blamed the epidemic on the French "licensed plunderers of the Ocean," adding that "if particular men had done their duty; and had not betrayed more indulgence to French cruizers, than genuine friendship for this city," the disease would have been averted.[23] Federalist charges fed a growing Francophobia. "AMOR PATRIAE" warned Philadelphians not to trust the city's benevolent French physicians. Persistent rumors that the wells had been contaminated preparatory to a French invasion led to threats of mob violence against the hapless refugees.[24]

Although the Federalists talked of closing all trade with the French islands, they seemed far more anxious to arouse public suspicion of the French and the Republicans than to create any precedent for a government embargo on commerce. Indeed, the Federalist merchants feared that localism was part of a Republican conspiracy to discredit Philadelphia and all large commercial centers and to force relocation of the capital in a rural setting. Richard Peters warned Timothy Pickering against Rush's doctrine on 22 October: "His Assertion that the Philadelphia Hot beds produced this deadly Plant is . . . a mischievous Opinion . . . and will be eagerly caught at by the Anti-Philadelphians. Stifle this Brat if you can."[25] Rush noted the result by 28 October: "A new clamor has been excited against me in which many citizens take a part. I have asserted that the yellow fever was generated in our city. This assertion they say will destroy the character of Philadelphia for healthiness, and drive Congress from it."[26] John Beale Bordley wrote an importationist pamphlet for the admitted purpose of convincing Congress to remain in Philadelphia. Federalist editor John Fenno worried that the domestic origin theory would "not only render multitudes uneasy and interrupt the usual course of business, but injure the interest and reputation of the city in several respects."[27]

Such political fears could easily distort medical objectivity. "Is there a city in the world," asked Levi Hollingsworth, "kept cleaner than Philadelphia?" The College of Physicians answered flatly, "No possible improvement with respect to water or ventilation can make our situation more eligible"—this at a time when Philadelphia had no sewage system, no fresh water supply, and no provision for regular garbage disposal![28]

Republicans did attack large cities as unhealthy, and Jefferson later expressed confidence that the "yellow fever will discourage the growth of great cities in our nation."[29] Yet most Republicans protested that they wanted not to destroy commercial cities but to preserve them through sanitary reform.[30] Federalist fears of a plot to move the capital also proved groundless. In the debates over whether or not Congress could legally meet elsewhere to avoid the fever, the Republicans, for strict constructionist reasons, favored convening in Philadelphia.[31]

The Federalist endorsement of importation proved to be a very effective and popular position as the idea of a native American plague irritated a highly sensitive patriotic nerve. Rush noted that "Loathsome and dangerous diseases have been considered by all nations as of foreign extraction."[32] Importationists made much of the widely held feeling that independent America was the New Eden. Reaching the farthest extreme of this argument, one importationist asserted in 1799 that the doctrine of domestic fevers was "treason," perhaps hoping that the Alien and Sedition Acts gave the Federalists the power to deport foreign diseases along with foreign agitators.[33]

The people of Philadelphia urged their officials to agree on specific actions to prevent the return of yellow fever, but the political implications of the issue made adoption of any single course of action unacceptable. Thus, immediately following the 1793 epidemic, Pennsylvania and other threatened states undertook *both* quarantine and sanitary reform projects. Simple political compromise provided a way around the bitter medical deadlock.[34] Considering the state of medical knowledge in 1793, the imposition of a political settlement may well have been the best result that could have been expected.

In 1793, the division between medicine and theology was still young. Not everyone in Philadelphia believed the cause of the plague was strictly medical; rather, the wrath of the Deity appeared to many as manifest in the fever, and before the debate over the epidemic had ended, theology, like medicine, had become enmeshed in political developments. The devout saw most early American diseases, such as cholera and typhoid, as punishment for the individual sins of vicious immigrants and slothful poor. Unlike these diseases, though, yellow fever was spread not by poor individual hygiene but by infected mosquitoes which could and did bite high and low with complete republican egalitarianism. Some physicians even declared that blacks and the West Indian immigrants were more immune than respectable white Philadelphians. At any rate, the pious saw the yellow fever as a communal punishment rather than as retribution against individual sinners.[35]

The issue that remained, of course, was to identify and root out those communal transgressions which had provoked the pestilence. With no shortage of suggestions as to where the country was going astray, the Republicans first gave political content to the religious debate. At the very height of the plague, Freneau devoted front page coverage to a series of articles and letters which pointed to the pride and vanity of the communal leaders as the major transgression. Mathew Carey joined in the attack. And Benjamin Rush, the Enlightenment man of science, commented in retrospect, "I agree with you in deriving our physical calamities from moral causes. . . . We ascribe all the attributes of the Deity to the name of General Washington. It is considered by our citizens as the bulwark of our nation. God would cease to be what He is, if he did not visit us for these things."[36]

Federalists too put the religious issue in political harness. An official thanksgiving-fast sermon by the Reverend William Smith linked the pestilence with French immorality and with the "wild principles and restless conduct of their partisans here, impatient of all rule and authority."[37] Connecticut Senator Chauncey Goodrich saw the divine anger resulting from Republican adoration of Genêt, while Alexander Graydon recalled the "state of parties in the summer of 1793, when the metropolis of Pennsylvania, then resounding with unhallowed orgies at the dismal butcheries in France, was visited with a calamity which had much the appearance which heaven sometimes sends to purify the heart."[38]

A peculiar coincidence gave added depth to these speculations, for the fever had miraculously appeared just as Philadelphia completed construction of what one Republican termed its "Synagogue for Satan"—the city's new Chestnut Street Theatre. Many in Revolutionary America saw the theater as an extremely complex negative symbol, part bordello and part palace. The new theater, with fluted marble columns and pure golden ornaments, was indeed palatial.[39] While a few Republicans like Swanwick owned stock in the theater company, the major backers were prominent Federalists.[40] They in turn tried to portray opposition to the theater as a Republican scheme to subvert private property. One Francophobe detected the same "rigourous enthusiasm" which spawned the French Revolution motivating the foes of the drama. Opponents of the stage did appeal to Anglophobic, antimonarchical, and Republican imagery to justify their cause, although not all Republicans were antitheater.[41]

Philadelphia's embattled defenders of public virtue had all but given up when the epidemic provided the ammunition for yet another crusade. Sixteen of the city's leading clergymen joined with the Quakers in petitioning the state to shut the new theater. "We conceive that the solemn intimations of Divine Providence in the late distressing calamity which has been experienced in this city, urge upon us in the most forcible manner the duty of reforming every thing which may be offensive to the Supreme Governor of the Universe." Devout Republicans found it significant that "the actors and retainers of the stage, who actually arrived here at a time when the fever raged with the utmost violence," were Englishmen.[42] The opponents of stage plays eventually lost their struggle, even with the arguments gained from the epidemic. The issue, however, helped strengthen the growing bond between Quakers and Republicans in Philadelphia.[43]

BLEEDING VS. BARK: THE CURE

Medical science today can do little more to cure a case of yellow fever than it could in 1793, a sobering fact that helps explain the continued controversy over the treatment of the disease long after the question of etiology had been shelved. The number of treatments attempted in the sheer desperation of the Philadelphia epidemic was astounding, yet the medical community rapidly split into two main schools. One favored the use of "stimulants"—quinine bark, wine, and cold baths—a method long used in both British and French West Indies. Opposing these "bark and wine murderers," a second group advocated the "new treatment" concocted by Dr. Rush, who believed it advisable to draw an amount of blood which we know today to be in excess of the quantity possessed by most people, and whose doses of mercury caused severe disfiguration of the teeth and skin. But by eighteenth-century standards his "experimental" approach appeared more advanced than the "traditional" bark cure.[44]

Many factors helped determine which doctors adopted what cure, not the least of which was chance. Rush himself tried the bark and wine method before his "discovery" but lost three of four patients. Another variable was the infamous, tangled infighting among Philadelphia physicians. Almost any medical opinion rendered by Benjamin Rush eventually drew the ridicule of Dr. William Shippen, the man Rush had hauled before a court martial over their disagreements in the Revolution.[45] Partisan differences were at first unimportant in a doctor's choice of a cure. True, Rush counted among his followers many ardent Republicans such as Dr. Leib, Dr. George Logan, the Quaker pacifist, Dr. Benjamin Say, and most of his former students. However, a large body of Republican "bark and wine doctors" included Hutchinson, Dr. Benjamin Smith Barton, and the French trained Bush Hill staff under Devèze and Girard. Republican bark doctors did learn the cure from the French refugees, while the Federalist Dr. Stevens and other non-Republican physicians adopted the procedure from the British or Dutch Islands, but their actual methods of treating patients were almost identical. Although it was inaccurate, many Philadelphians persisted in the conviction that there was a "Republican cure" and a "Federalist cure."[46]

The man initially responsible for politically polarizing this nonpartisan jumble was Alexander Hamilton. Seeing an opportunity to do a favor for an old friend, Hamilton published a glowing personal tribute to Dr. Stevens, attributing his own recovery to the bark and wine cure. In so doing, Hamilton could not resist a sneer at his old critic, Dr. Rush. Hamilton's tool, Secretary of War Henry Knox, followed, airing his thoughts on Rush a few days later. The local and national Federalist press took the cue and began a barrage of political-sounding attacks on Rush's cure, terminated only by the 1799 libel judgment against Cobbett. Fenno's unkind attempt to derive Rush's bloodletting from that of the French terror resulted in a libel action against him as well, but the case was never tried.[47]

By simply declaring long enough and loud enough that bark and wine was the Federalist cure, these editors were able to make a considerable political issue out of a basically nonpartisan dispute. Their appeal was meant to gain political support among the many users of the mild wine and quinine therapy while personally discrediting Rush. The political element in the attack on bleeding seemed obvious to Rush. "I think it probable that if the new remedies had been introduced by any other person than a decided Democrat and a friend of Madison and Jefferson, they would have met with less opposition from Colonel Hamilton," Rush complained. "Many of us," he later told General Horatio Gates, "have been forced to expiate our sacrifices in the cause of liberty by suffering every species of slander and perse-

cution. I ascribe the opposition to my remedies in the epidemic which desolated our city in 1793 chiefly to an unkind and resentful association of my
political principles with my medical character."[48] Rush did not deny the
Federalist charge that his cures were associated with his politics. Attacked
as a democrat, he replied as a democrat, hoping to rally Republican political
support for his medical views. Rush declared his cure the only truly egalitarian form of medicine in that it was easy to master and could be practiced by
anyone with little formal training. Putting his beliefs into practice, he
trained a group of free blacks as itinerant bleeders during the epidemic and
published "do-it-yourself" directions in the newspapers, actions which did
not endear him to the guardians of the professional mysteries any more than
to the Federalists. Rush declared it unnecessary "to send men educated in
colleges . . . to cure . . . pestilential disease," assuring his followers that
"men and even women may be employed for that purpose, who have not
perverted their reason by a servile attachment to any system of medicine."
"All that is necessary," he added, "might be taught to a boy or girl twelve
years old in a few hours."[49]

Rush also adopted the Federalists' derogatory identification of his cures
with the French Revolution, affirming "I am in the situation of The French
Republic surrounded and invaded by new as well as old enemies, without any
other allies." He went so far as to imply that the true treatment, no less than
the true politics, could be derived in good democratic fashion: "The people
rule here in medicine as well as government." The best cure could be decided
by the will of the majority. On 2 October, Rush wrote to Elias Boudinot that
"Colonel Hamilton's remedies are now as unpopular in our city as his funding
system is in Virginia or North Carolina."[50]

Public support of bark and wine by several prominent Federalists gave
credence to its reputation as the "Federalist cure." Rush, however, failed in
his attempt to rally the Republican leadership behind his "egalitarian" medicine. Prominent Republican leaders largely ignored the issue on which Republican physicians were themselves divided.

No clear political division over the issue of therapy actually existed, despite the highly publicized attempts of Hamilton and Rush to create such a
polarization. Republican "bark and wine" physicians denied that bleeding
was the Republican cure, but they could not compete for public attention with
the colorful and prolific Dr. Benjamin Rush. Many Republican "bark doctors"
were refugees, barred from political office and lacking public influence, and
Hutchinson's death deprived them of their most prominent and articulate
spokesman. The failure of "bark and wine" Republicans to counter the pub-
licity attracted by Hamilton and Rush made the cure of yellow fever seem a
clear cut party issue.[51] Moreover, the injection of politics into this medical
debate probably had some adverse side effects. The partisan taint of argu-

ments against mercury and bleeding delayed rejection of the Rush cure long after the medical evidence pointed to its inefficacy and danger.

TO FLEE OR NOT TO FLEE: THE CREDIT

The first days of the epidemic produced a mad scramble to escape town. Benjamin Rush warned all who could to leave the city; even his bitter rivals Drs. Shippen and Kuhn took his advice this time and quickly departed. The panic was so great that "many people thrust their parents into the streets, as soon as they complained of a headache."[52] Exceptions to the general exodus soon appeared, however. Most of the physicians stuck to their posts. Rush, following his discovery of a "cure," publicly advised everyone to remain in town. The French, familiar with the disease and trained to believe it noncontagious, did not flee. Many shopkeepers and middle-class merchants with no one to look after their affairs, and the poor with no place else to go, stayed as well. A handful of true philanthropists remained. As the epidemic wore on, observers noted that the leaders of each of these groups were often Republicans.[53]

Several Federalists did play major roles in the heroic relief work. Mayor Clarkson organized the citizens' committee while Samuel Coates and John Oldden headed a merchants' distribution organization which handled supplies for the mayor. Coates, an intimate of Rush and Girard, was nonetheless a Federalist and was often criticized by Girard for his Francophobia.[54] Levi Hollingsworth and Caspar W. Morris joined the merchants' group. Clement Humphreys, son of the ship-builder, remained at his post as a guardian of the poor. Three Federalist clergymen, William Smith, William White, and Robert Blackwell, also remained to comfort the ill. Although these nine men were the only identifiable Federalists at all involved in the organized relief work, an additional five, Jacob Hiltzheimer, Postmaster Timothy Pickering, ex-Postmaster Ebenezer Hazard, Congressman Thomas FitzSimmons, and John Stillé, chose not to join the organized effort but rendered important aid to their families and neighbors individually.[55]

Active Republicans, however, performed the greatest share of the work. Of the 18 men cited in the minutes as the leaders of the citizens' committee, nine were definitely Republicans, one was the brother of an ardent Republican, and seven could not be identified with either party. The mayor was the only Federalist. The Republican leaders of the committee were Vice-Chairman Samuel Wetherill, Secretary Caleb Lownes, Stephen Girard of Bush Hill, Israel Israel (orphans), Mathew Carey (printing), Jonathan Dickinson Sergeant (counsel), James Sharswood (accounts), James Kerr (orphans), and John Connelly (accounts). Treasurer Thomas Wistar was the brother of Republican Dr. Caspar Wistar.[56] The other committeemen were Andrew Adgate (at large), Peter Helm of Bush Hill, Daniel Offley (at large), Joseph Inskeep (at large), John Letchworth (orphans), Samuel Benge (burials), and Henry Deforest (supplies).

Three of the four members of the key correspondence committee which ran the Democratic Society were leaders in fighting the fever. Two, Hutchinson and Jonathan Dickinson Sergeant, lost their lives while caring for the sick. The third was Dr. Leib, who had charge of Bush Hill in the first chaotic days of its existence. Alexander B. Dallas, the fourth member, claimed with some justification that his state office required him to follow the state government to its exile in Germantown.[57] At least 17 men listed as active in the Democratic Society played major roles in aiding the sick. Israel Israel directed the relief and orphanage work of the committee. Well known in Philadelphia for his Revolutionary War exploits and for his antifederalism, Israel was treasurer of the Democratic Society. The president of the society, David Rittenhouse, went on call with his nephew Dr. Barton, arranging for free treatment of the poor. After the death of his son-in-law Sergeant, Rittenhouse left town briefly, but returned before the end of the epidemic to resume his work.[58]

The Quaker Dr. George Logan was an ardent Democrat who had left both medicine and Philadelphia in 1781. Returning now from his retirement at Stenton near Germantown, he served as the committee's inspector at Bush Hill, from where he reported to the world the incredible efforts of the managers, "Citizens Girard and Helm." The one-eyed merchant Girard, who almost alone turned Bush Hill from a pesthouse to a hospital, was also active in the Democratic organization.[59] The labors of Dr. Rush, who formally joined the society in early 1794, were comparable to those of Girard. Visiting hundreds of patients while ill himself, Rush stuck to his post even after the death of his sister. Also members of the Democratic group were John Connelly and James Kerr of the citizens' committee; George Forepaugh, Jeremiah Paul, William Robinson, Sr., James Swaine, and William Watkins of the merchants' committee; volunteer John Barker; and John Swanwick, owner of the committee's orphanage. Others of Republican persuasion cited for their roles were aldermen Hilary Baker and John Barclay, and merchants' committeeman Caspar Snyder.[60]

Among Philadelphia newspapers, only Republican Andrew Brown's *Federal Gazette* appeared throughout the epidemic, keeping the remaining citizens in touch with the relief workers.[61] Freneau, who vowed to publish for as long as possible, held on longer than any editor except Brown. The *National Gazette* last appeared on 16 October, a victim of financial losses rather than of editorial dereliction. His work ended, Freneau did not flee the city but remained until mid-December.[62]

The list of Republican heroes also included Frenchmen. In addition to Devèze, all four physicians' aides and most of the staff at Bush Hill were French. The French specialist in tropical medicine, Citizen Robert, hearing of the epidemic while en route to France, rushed to Philadelphia from Boston in what one writer termed a "confirmation of the sincere attachment of the French patriots, to the truly republican Americans!" The largest individual contribution to the relief fund came from Citizen Genêt. Even "THE RE-PUBLICAN SEAMEN OF FRANCE" got involved, forming Philadelphia's only intact fire company during the epidemic. Freneau credited them with saving the city from the fate of London.[63]

While Republicans dominated the relief work, Federalists often joined the ranks of the refugees, not necessarily from cowardice, as Republicans charged, but rather because of their belief in importation and contagion. No prominent importationist leaders of either party stayed in Philadelphia. The one anticontagionist Federalist official remained; the one importationist Republican fled. Illustrative of the disappearance of Federalists was the case of the Dutch Minister, Francis Van Berkle, who believed himself ill. Since Dr. Stevens had left for New York, Hamilton (from his refuge in Albany) suggested that the minister consult Oliver Wolcott on the use of bark and wine. The minister soon discovered that Wolcott too was gone. Tired of looking for someone to instruct him in the "Federalist cure," Van Berkle was treated by Rush and recovered.[64]

It appeared that the Republicans would receive high praise for their efforts. Benjamin Rush "is become the darling of the common people and his humane fortitude and exertions will render him deservedly dear," noted one observer.[65] Bravery and leadership make popular American campaign fare, and the Republicans were not slow to present their political bill for services rendered. Among the first to make an issue of bravery was Jefferson, whose Revolutionary War record had recently come under unkind Federalist scrutiny. His scornful cut at Hamilton as the Treasury Secretary prepared to flee is considered by Dumas Malone to have been Jefferson's most vicious political remark. "His family think him in danger," wrote Jefferson, "and he puts himself so by his excessive alarm. He has been miserable several days before from a firm persuasion he should catch it. A man as timid as he is on the water, as timid on horseback, as timid in sickness, would be a phenomenon if his courage of which he has the reputation in military occasions were genuine. His friends, who have not seen him, suspect it is only an autumnal fever he has." Jefferson also attacked Henry Knox, who had already fled, but after waiting to make sure Hamilton had really gone first, Jefferson himself left town over a week ahead of his planned departure.[66]

Freneau took over the task of castigating the "deserters." His poem, "Orlando's Flight," ridiculed the fugitives:

On prancing steed, with spunge at nose,
From town behold Orlando fly;
Camphor and Tar where'er he goes

132

Th' infected shafts of death defy—
    Safe in an atmosphere of stink,
    No doctor gets Orlando's chink.

Freneau also implied it was greed that made the fugitives so anxious to preserve themselves. Speaking of the afterworld, he concluded:

Monarchs are there of little note,
And Caesar wears a ragged coat.
. . . .
Blame not Orlando if he fled,—
So little's got by being dead.[67]

The last evacuees had not yet returned when a special election brought the
heroism issue to the fore. State Senator Samuel Powel, Philadelphia's beloved
Revolutionary War mayor, had died of the fever. On 12 December, a Republican meeting put forth the name of Israel Israel for Powel's seat. Israel's platform was simple and direct. He was "a gentleman whose philanthropy on a late
melancholy occasion is well known, and whose firm and steady attachment to
the people will, it is hoped, bring forth the united suffrages of the citizens in his
favour."[68] The Federalist response came swiftly. The day after the Israel nomination, Fenno revealed a move to draft Mayor Clarkson as the Federalist choice.
In an attempt to outdo the Republicans, Clarkson's backers asserted that "gratitude demands a particular tribute of acknowledgement to him for his assiduity,
and perseverance in relieving the distresses of our fellow citizens during the
calamity from which we have just emerged."[69] Clarkson, however, was content
to be mayor, and the nomination went instead to William Bingham, the extremely wealthy associate of the powerful Willing-Morris partnership. Bingham
had followed the progress of the fever from his New Jersey shore retreat. The
actual management of his campaign, however, was placed in the hands of relief
workers John Oldden and John Stillé. Their efforts apparently countered the
appeal of Israel's candidacy, and Bingham won the 19 December contest by a
three to two margin.[70]

The return of the "deserters" further complicated Republican use of the
heroism issue. While many of the Federalists had fled the fever, most of the
evacuees were not Federalists. One-third of all Philadelphians had left, and
the majority of the rest remained hidden behind locked doors, venturing out
only for necessities. Their initial gratitude toward the members of the committee was mingled with a good deal of shame, guilt, and envy. As one per-
ceptive reviewer noted in commenting on Mathew Carey's account of the
epidemic, "To panegyrize our contemporaries, without attracting censure on
ourselves, requires a very delicate hand."[71] The Republicans realized that a

campaign based solely on praising their own heroics while damning the opposition's defections was politically unwise. They usually attempted to temper their attacks by expressing sympathy with the difficulties encountered by the fugitives, many of whom had been brutally repulsed by the panicked citizens of neighboring cities.[72]

The returnees meanwhile countered criticism with charges of their own, terming the epidemic a "doctors' harvest." The citizens' committee was attacked as too expensive and as growing insolent with power. "Unless the Committee feel *tickled* with their employment," wrote one critic, "they ought to surrender it to the Guardians of the poor, who are competent to the service, and who will perform it at a *much less expence* and *with far less state*." Rush's black bleeders were easy targets for Federalist charges of profiteering. Actually, the committee and most physicians offered free medical service to the poor, while Rush even distributed free mercury. Yet the boast of Rush's student, Dr. Mease, that the fever had made his fortune for life, and the activities of Samuel Wetherill, whose drug business took precedence over his committee duties, gave the charges just enough credibility to undermine the Republican appeal to public gratitude.[73] A common complaint charged the committeemen with usurping powers reserved for the traditional political elite. "The bulk of them," wrote one resentful critic, "are scarcely known beyond the smoke of their own chimnies."[74] Further, many Philadelphians simply wished to forget the entire painful scene as quickly as possible. The heroes of the epidemic were living reminders of the horror and the suffering. "If the disease has disappeared as it no doubt has, every memento of its existence should disappear with it, that the citizens may once more enjoy repose."[75]

Despite the strenuous efforts of the party organization, Republican heroism was a complete flop as a political issue. A 1797 election in which Israel Israel had defeated Federalist Benjamin Morgan was invalidated when Morgan claimed his backers had been disenfranchised by holding the election while the Federalists were "driven from their homes" by the epidemic of that year. With the fleeing Federalists safely home again, the hapless Israel lost the second election despite heavy contributions from Girard and Sharswood.[76]

CONCLUSION: HEALTH AS A POLITICAL ISSUE

The yellow fever struck a Federalist Philadelphia in 1793 and left both local and national Federalist rule considerably strengthened. For one thing, the epidemic seriously weakened the national Republican organization. The deaths of Hutchinson and Sergeant eliminated two of the four men responsible for creating and directing new Democratic Society branches. Years later, John Adams declared that these two deaths alone saved the nation from an imminent revolution.[77] The collapse of the *National Gazette* under the financial strain of the epidemic created another void which Bache's *Aurora* could not immediately fill. Even the little-noted death of Citizen Dupont, the French consul, had its political effect, leaving France's critical relations with the United States in the hands of a vice-consul for months until the arrival of a replacement for Genêt.

In issues as well as institutions the Federalists gained, at least in the short run. The Republicans were unable to convert their heavy organizational losses into an effective sympathy vote. By denying any local source of the pestilence, the Federalists won much national chauvinist and local booster support, while their espousal of importationism heightened American Francophobia. In addition, the Federalists managed to identify their opponents with Benjamin Rush's advocacy of a dangerous and controversial remedy. Although Philadelphia Republicans found some additional Quaker support in the theater issue, the national party gained at best a minor new point against large cities.[78]

More important, the epidemic served to introduce new issues and attract new supporters to the two developing parties, thereby extending and broadening the base of the new party system. This development was sometimes local in its origins, as in the debate over the cause of the fever, where the already politically polarized local controversy introduced issues that the national politicians adopted and used. In other issues, such as the bleeding *v.* bark debate, a nonpolarized initial conflict had political meaning imposed from the outside by the intervention of national leaders. Furthermore, the process of giving political significance to social issues was highly selective. The issue which seemed logically closest to politics was that of courage and leadership, but despite the efforts of the local antagonists and the party organization, human feelings of gratitude provided too flimsy a foundation on which to build a political platform.

Neither the risks of disease nor the costs of fighting it are evenly distributed in American society. This inequality, resulting from both biological and social conditions, creates the potential for political division over almost all aspects of public health. But not every health issue actually produces a political conflict. Interest groups overlap in complex ways. Consider, for example, the dilemma facing Federalist merchants, who would gain from a quarantine of the French islands, but simultaneously would suffer from any increase in the rigor of quarantines in general.

Political influence in late eighteenth-century medicine did not always signify irresponsible meddling. Political compromise permitted concerted public action to fight future epidemics at a time when medical opinion seemed hopelessly deadlocked, although the political significance of the potentially lethal Rush "cure" helped assure its continued use, needlessly endangering the lives of patients.

Finally, not everyone was willing to be drawn into partisan debate over a medical question. Expressing the hope that the next epidemic might be met by the united efforts of "all parties" in the City of Brotherly Love, an anonymous satirist poked fun at both the Federalist and Republican views of the fever:

> Be patient ye vivid sons of mercury with the medical baptisms of your *cold bath brethren*. For had that therapeutic process been tried under the cataract of Niagara, no body can tell the wonders which might have been produced by it . . .
>
> Cease ye yellow fever heroes to censure, those of your brethren whose delicacy of nerves and previous engagements called them suddenly crochet and forceps a la main to Nootka Sound, to catch Otters and Beavers. Be assured, important discoveries have been made by the Jaunt.
>
> Lend a Kind ear to the graduates of Montpelier, who inform you that the late disease arose from the burying grounds in the heart of your city, since in France they never bury the dead under Churches, but in balloons high up in the air.[79]
>
> Ye learned and long robed sons of Esculapius, pity and pardon poor Absolam [sic] Jones and Richard Allen,[80] two sable Ethiopians, who being ignorant of the Greek and Latin Languages, were under the necessity of curing their patients *in English*.[81]

But neither the political nor the medical debates would be silenced so simply.

AFTERWORD

The quarter-century since I began writing this article witnessed an outpouring of scholarship on the history of disease in general and on yellow fever in particular. Although prior to the present volume surprisingly little of this new work studied the wave of yellow fever epidemics that struck northern American cities from 1793 to the 1820s, the new scholarship requires that this article be updated in four main areas.

First, race may have played a bigger role in both the medical and the political history than I originally recognized. The article notes that many physicians of 1793 thought blacks were more immune than whites, but it implicitly discounts the modern value of such observations by claiming that infected mosquitoes actually bit everyone equally. The implication that yellow fever was color blind has since been sharply challenged. Kenneth Kiple and Virginia Kiple argued that in late-nineteenth-century epidemics, proportionately fewer blacks than whites died of yellow fever.[82] Like Phillip Lapsansky's observation in this volume, Kiple and Kiple admit that blacks and whites both had high disease rates, and that blacks suffered many deaths. But Kiple and Kiple argue that some unknown, perhaps biological, factor produced a racial difference in death rates. In the 1793 epidemic, taking into account Lapsansky's calculation that whites fled infected regions of Philadelphia at much higher rates than blacks, the death rate for whites as a proportion of the population remaining in town in 1793 may have been as much as one-third higher than the death rate for remaining blacks.

However, even if such a racial difference in mortality actually existed in 1793, it may not have been due to genetics. The difference could also have been due to underreporting of black deaths or underestimating the number of Philadelphia blacks from endemic regions like Haiti. Or it could have resulted from the group protection native-born blacks might have received from living among a concentrated group of previously immune immigrants, or from differences in exposure to mosquitoes due to residence, occupation, dress, or diet.

Modern confirmation of a racial difference in death rates would have no impact on the validity of my main point, which concerned 1793 perceptions rather than current evaluations of their accuracy. But my comment about egalitarian mosquitoes now appears both irrelevant and simplistic.

More importantly, I missed the chance to draw a revealing comparison between white and black volunteers, each of whom failed to convert their heroism into significant political gains. The white Republican mechanics who served as volunteers were ignored by the city's Federalist elite and were resented by the many voters who had fled, but their political exclusion was less severe than the scornful ingratitude shown to Richard Allen's and Absalom Jones' black followers. Considering the two together shows that racial differences as well as class similarities played a role in the political rejection of both the black and white heroes. And while Jones and Allen concentrated their criticism on white volunteers like Mathew Carey, the two groups had many economic and political similarities. Both Carey and the black leaders wrote their pamphlets in part because they felt their followers had been denied political recognition for their contributions by the white Federalist elite.

Second, on many of the debates over yellow fever the medical sides were not as sharply dichotomized as this paper implies. For example, I presented the battle over therapies as a stark choice: heroic doses of bleeding and purging versus supportive doses of chinchona bark and wine. I found that even if only these two therapies are considered, politics fails to explain which doctors followed which therapies. The noisy rivalry between Rush and Hamilton created a widely-accepted but erroneous impression that bleeding and purging was the treatment favored by most Republican doctors. But I missed an even larger point. As Worth Estes points out in this volume, bleeding and bark were hardly the only remedies available, nor were they mutually exclusive. The therapeutic reality was much more complex and eclectic. The same political debate that created the false image that all Republicans backed Rush's cures also created the false impression that there were only two incompatible treatment options.

Likewise, the medical debate between importationists and local origin supporters was not as dichotomized as I implied. Recent scholarship emphasizes the variety of intermediary positions in eighteenth- and nineteenth-century etiology, including one theory that disease might require both an imported "seed" and a receptive local "soil" in which to grow.[83] As a result, it was an overstatement to claim that the eventual decision to pursue both quarantine and sanitation was a purely political resolution, a pragmatic compromise of logically incompatible medical positions. Though that picture is largely correct, there were medical as well as political grounds for the outcome.

Third, this paper begins with the claim that political factors influenced medicine primarily at times of medical uncertainty. That assertion conflicts with the ending, in which I argue that medicine and public health are inherently partly political. On reflection, I would now emphasize the second point, and amend the first to say that medical controversies simply make medicine's inherently political and ethical dimensions easier to see.

Finally, while the reception of this paper among medical historians has been gratifying, when I wrote it I was aiming at a different audience. I had hoped to demonstrate the links between political and social-cultural history. Perhaps partly as a result of the long split between them, both political and social-cultural historians have largely overlooked or seemingly misread the point of the piece.[84] But the gap between these two camps has recently been bridged by social-cultural historians eager to "bring the state back" into their work. The history of government efforts in public health should occupy a prominent place in this new cultural history of the state.

NOTES

1. J. H. Powell, *Bring Out Your Dead: The Great Plague of Yellow Fever in Philadelphia in 1793* (Philadelphia: University of Pennsylvania Press, 1949), pp. 1–64; Charles E. A. Winslow, *The Conquest of Epidemic Disease: A Chapter in the History of Ideas* (Princeton: Princeton University Press, 1943), p. 198.

2. Powell, *Bring Out Your Dead*, pp. 8–12, 219, 232. The exact number of deaths is unknown. The figure 4,040, derived from burial lists, includes deaths from all causes in the city but does not include the many fever victims buried elsewhere. The burial lists are appended to Mathew Carey, *A Short Account of the Malignant Fever, . . .* 4th ed. (Philadelphia: Mathew Carey, 1794). See also Richard H. Shryock, *Medicine and Society in America, 1660–1860* (New York: New York University Press, 1960), pp. 82, 108.

3. Powell, *Bring Out Your Dead*, pp. 242–243.

4. Erwin H. Ackerknecht, "Anticontagionism Between 1821 and 1867," *Bulletin of the History of Medicine* 26 (1948): 562–593. An opposing view is J.B. Blake, "Yellow Fever in Eighteenth-Century America," *Bulletin of the New York Academy of Medicine* 44 (1968): 681.

5. Eugene P. Link, *Democratic-Republican Societies, 1790–1800* (New York: Columbia University Press, 1942); Harry M. Tinkcom, *The Republicans and Federalists in Pennsylvania, 1790–1801: A Study in National Stimulus and Local Response* (Harrisburg: Pennsylvania Historical and Museum Commission, 1950).

6. Frances S. Childs, *French Refugee Life in the United States, 1790–1800: An American Chapter of the French Revolution* (Baltimore: Johns Hopkins University Press, 1940), pp. 22, 103, 142–143, 159.

7. A general picture of the events and mechanisms of party development may be found in Joseph Charles, *The Origins of the American Party System* (New York: Harper and Row, 1956); Noble E. Cunningham, Jr., *The Jeffersonian Republicans: The Formation of Party Organization, 1789–1801* (Chapel Hill: University of North Carolina Press, 1957); Richard Hofstadter, *The Idea of a Party System: The Rise of Legitimate Opposition in the United States, 1780–1840* (Berkeley and Los Angeles: University of California Press, 1969); and Richard P. McCormick, *The Second American Party System: Party Formation in the Jacksonian Era* (Chapel Hill: University of North Carolina Press, 1966).

8. Winslow, *Epidemic Disease*, pp. 195, 200, 231. Related to, but distinct from, the etiology question was the problem of contagion. Almost all importationists believed the fever contagious, but advocates of a local origin differed over whether it could become contagious after appearing. For examples, see David Nassy, *Observations on the Cause, Nature, and Treatment of the Epidemic Disorder Prevalent in Philadelphia* (Philadelphia: Printed by Parker and Co., for M. Carey, 1793), p. 13; Benjamin Rush, *An Enquiry Into the Origin of the Late Epidemic Fever in Philadelphia* (Philadelphia: Mathew Carey, 1793), p. 14; Benjamin S. Barton, "On Yellow Fever," n.d. [1806?], Benjamin Smith Barton Papers, Delafield Collection, American Philosophical Society, Philadelphia.

9. Powell, *Bring Out Your Dead*, pp. 43–44; Carey, *Short Account*, p. 12; Benjamin Rush, *An Account of the Bilious Remitting Yellow Fever . . .* (Philadelphia: Printed by Thomas Dobson, 1794); *Dictionary of American Biography*, s.v. "Hutchinson, James"; Jean Devèze, *An Enquiry into, and Observations upon, the Causes and Effects of the Epidemic Disease* (Philadelphia: Printed by Parent, 1794), p. 16; Powell, *Bring Out Your Dead*, pp. 36–44. On the importance of the correspondence committee, see Edward Ford, *David Rittenhouse: Astronomer-Patriot, 1732–1796* (Philadelphia: University of Pennsylvania Press, 1946), p. 190.

10. Records of the College of Physicians, 1 (1787–1812), p. 175, 19 November 1793, College of Physicians of Philadelphia; Rush, *Account*, p. 146; Adam Kuhn, Yellow Fever Manuscripts (1794), p. 6, College of Physicians of Philadelphia, Philadelphia; Stacey B. Day, ed., *Edward Stevens: Gastric Physiologist, Physician and American Statesman* (Montreal and Cincinnati: Cultural and Educational Productions, 1969); William Currie, *A Treatise on the Synochus Icteroides, or Yellow Fever . . .* (Philadelphia: Printed by Thomas Dobson, 1794), pp. 1, 67, 84; Currie, *An Impar-*

tial Review of That Part of Dr. Rush's Late Publication . . . In Which His Opinion Is Shewn to be Erroneous; the Importation of the Disease Established; and the Wholesomeness of the City Vindicated (Philadelphia: Printed by Thomas Dobson, 1794), pp. 6–14.

11. Rush, *Account*, p. 146; *Independent Gazetteer* (Philadelphia), 22 January 1794; Benjamin S. Barton to Thomas Pennant, 11 April 1794, Barton Papers. Later epidemics in 1797 and 1798 introduced some blurring of party lines. By 1797, Republican Dr. Caspar Wistar had definitely joined the importationists. See College of Physicians of Philadelphia, *Facts and Observations Relative to the Nature and Origin of the Pestilential Fever . . .* (Philadelphia: Printed for Thomas Dobson, 1798), pp. 43, 52; Samuel D. Gross, ed., *Lives of Eminent American Physicians and Surgeons of the Nineteenth Century* (Philadelphia: Lindsay and Blakiston, 1861), pp. 134–135; College of Physicians Records, 1, pp. 216, 225, 250. The political allegiance of Dr. William Shippen, Jr., is uncertain. An importationist, he chaired a largely Republican town meeting in 1795 but also appeared in the rolls of the Federalist marching society. See *Independent Gazetteer*, 30 November 1793, 25 July 1795; and General Roll of McPherson's Blues, Hollingsworth Manuscripts, Business Papers Miscellaneous, undated, Historical Society of Pennsylvania, Philadelphia. An unlikely suggestion was made that Shippen did not know who was behind the 1795 meeting, "thus committing himself as a puppet to be moved at the pleasure of very bungling artists." *Gazette of the United States* (Philadelphia), 25 July 1795. Dr. Charles Caldwell continued to champion localism even after his 1796 conversion to Federalism, but in 1793 he was loyal to both the politics and the medicine of Benjamin Rush. See Charles Caldwell, *Autobiography* (Philadelphia: Lippincott, Grambo, and Co., 1855), pp. 174, 182, 254, 267, 278; Caldwell to James Hutchinson, 1 August 1793, Hutchinson Papers, American Philosophical Society.

12. Benjamin Rush, *Medical Inquiries and Observations* (Philadelphia: Printed and Sold by Prichard and Hall, 1789); and Carl Binger, *Revolutionary Doctor: Benjamin Rush, 1746–1813* (New York: Norton, 1966), p. 228.

13. Rush, for one, expected just such deference from former students. See *Letters of Benjamin Rush*, ed. L. H. Butterfield, 2 vols. (Princeton: American Philosophical Society, 1951), 2: 681.

14. Powell feels Hutchinson was "obviously confused." *Bring Out Your Dead*, p. 43. See also n. 23 below.

15. "Pestilence," quoted in Powell, *Bring Out Your Dead*, p. xxvi.

16. *National Gazette* (Philadelphia), 23 September 1793.

17. Thomas Jefferson to James Madison, 1 September 1793, in *The Writings of Thomas Jefferson*, ed. Andrew A. Lipscomb and Albert E. Bergh, 20 vols. (Washington, D.C.: Issued Under the Auspices of the Thomas Jefferson Memorial Association of the United States, 1903), 9: 214–215; *Federal Gazette* (Philadelphia), 17, 21, and 28 December 1793; *Gazette of the United States*, 18 December 1793. Democratic Society leader Israel Israel requested the city to dig sewers following the epidemic. Israel to Clarkson, 29 January 1794, Philadelphia Streets and Alleys Manuscripts, Historical Society of Pennsylvania.

18. For Fenno, see Nathan Goodman, *Benjamin Rush: Physician and Citizen, 1746–1813* (Philadelphia: University of Pennsylvania Press, 1934), p. 198; for Wolcott, see Charles Francis Jenkins, *Washington in Germantown . . .* (Philadelphia: W.J.

Campbell, 1905), p. 76; for Willing and Chew, see College of Physicians of Philadelphia, *Additional Facts and Observations Relative to the Nature and Origin of the Pestilential Fever* (Philadelphia: Printed by A. Bartram for Thomas Dobson, 1806), pp. 10, 11; for Hollingsworth, see "An Old Resident" [Hollingsworth] to David Claypoole, Hollingsworth MSS; for Bordley, see J. B. Bordley, *Yellow Fever* (Philadelphia: Printed by Charles Cist [?], 1794); for Hazard see "Hazard Letters," Massachusetts Historical Society, *Collections*, 5th ser., 3 (1877), p. 338, and Powell, *Bring Out Your Dead*, p. 86; for White, see Bird Wilson, *Memoir of the Life of the Right Reverend William White, D.D.,* . . . (Philadelphia: J. Kay Jun. and Brother, 1839), pp. 158, 288; for Johnson, see Benjamin Johnson, *Account of the Rise, Progress, and Termination of the Malignant Fever* (Philadelphia: Printed and Sold by Benjamin Johnson, 1793), p. 5.

19. Lewis Saul Benjamin [Lewis Melville], *The Life and Letters of William Cobbett in England and America, Based Upon Hitherto Unpublished Family Papers* (New York: John Lane Co., 1913), pp. 85–87.

20. For Mifflin, see Powell, *Bring Out Your Dead*, pp. 52–53, Samuel Hazard et al., eds., *Pennsylvania Archives*, 4th ser., 4 (Harrisburg: Harrisburg Publishing Co., 1900), pp. 264–269, and Tinkcom, *Republicans and Federalists*, pp. 72, 112, 219–220; for Bache, see Donald H. Stewart, *The Opposition Press of the Federalist Period* (Albany: State University of New York Press, 1969), p. 137; for Carey, see Mathew Carey, *Observations on Dr. Rush's Enquiry into the Origin of the Late Epidemic Fever in Philadelphia* (Philadelphia: Mathew Carey, 1793), and Carey, *Short Account*, p. 67.

21. Charles W. Upham, *The Life of Timothy Pickering*, 4 vols. (Boston: Little, Brown, and Co., 1873), 3: 56, 62. Some Federalists from rival cities, such as Harrisburg's Alexander Graydon, encouraged the idea that Philadelphia was an unhealthy place. Alexander Graydon, *Memoirs of a Life* (Harrisburg: Printed by John Wyeth, 1811), pp. 336–338. However, most Federalist merchants in New York, Baltimore, and Trenton remained importationists, leading the local efforts to cut off the trade of their stricken rival. See *General Advertiser* (Philadelphia), 18, 20, and 23 September 1793; and James Weston Livingood, *The Philadelphia-Baltimore Trade Rivalry 1780–1860* (Harrisburg: Pennsylvania Historical and Museum Commission, 1947). Even anticontagionist New York Federalist Noah Webster believed this Philadelphia epidemic contagious. Noah Webster, *A Collection of Papers on the Subject of Bilious Fevers* (New York: Printed by Hopkins, Webb, and Co., 1796), p. 233.

22. Harry Emerson Wildes, *Lonely Midas: The Story of Stephen Girard* (New York: Farrar, and Rinehart, Inc., 1943), pp. 121, 126; Albert J. Gares, "Stephen Girard's West Indian Trade, 1789–1812," *Pennsylvania Magazine of History and Biography* 72 (1948): 316; J. Thomas Scharf and Thompson Westcott, *History of Philadelphia, 1609–1884*, 3 vols. (Philadelphia: L.H. Everts, 1884), 1: 493.

23. Johnson, *Account*, pp. 5, 9; *Dunlap's American Daily Advertiser* (Philadelphia), 20 December 1793; Rush, *Account*, p. 147. Leib and others defended Hutchinson against the charges raised by the College. *General Advertiser*, 30 November, 10 December 1793.

24. *Independent Gazetteer*, 14 December 1793; Henry D. Biddle, ed., *Extracts from the Journal of Elizabeth Drinker* (Philadelphia: J.B. Lippincott Co., 1889), p. 193.

25. Richard Peters to Timothy Pickering, 22 October 1793, Timothy Pickering Papers, Massachusetts Historical Society, Boston, quoted in *Rush Letters*, 2: 729–730. Pickering may have shown the letter to Rush. Fearing government restrictions on trade, one Federalist importationist appealed to the benevolence of the merchants and ship captains to impose a voluntary quarantine. "A Philadelphian," in *Occasional Essays on the Yellow Fever* . . . (Philadelphia: Printed by John Ormond, 1800), pp. 8–11, 13.

26. Benjamin Rush to Julia Rush, 28 October 1793, in *Rush Letters*, 2: 729.

27. Goodman, *Benjamin Rush*, p. 198; Bordley, *Yellow Fever*, p. 1; and Blake, "Yellow Fever," p. 682.

28. "An Old Resident" to Claypoole, Hollingsworth MSS; and College of Physicians, *Facts and Observations*, p. 24.

29. Jefferson to Rush, 23 September 1800, quoted in Charles N. Glaab, *The American City: A Documentary History* (Homewood, Ill.: Dorsey Press, 1963), p. 52.

30. For example, *Federal Gazette*, 6, 21 December 1793; John Redman Coxe Letters on the Yellow Fever [1794], p. 139, College of Physicians of Philadelphia; Joseph McFarland, "The Epidemic of Yellow Fever in 1793 and Its Influence Upon Dr. Benjamin Rush," *Medical Life* 36 (1929): 468. Both sides in the medical split claimed to be the true friends of commerce. Blake, "Yellow Fever," p. 681.

31. Powell, *Bring Out Your Dead*, pp. 260–263. Constitutional principles did not limit the state's power to move its own capital out of Philadelphia in 1799 as a result of the yellow fever. Scharf and Westcott, *Philadelphia*, 1: 501.

32. Rush, *Account*, p. 147.

33. College of Physicians, *Facts and Observations*, pp. 15–16; *Rush Letters*, 2: 798; Hazard et al., eds., *Pennsylvania Archives*, 4th ser., 4: 269.

34. Blake, "Yellow Fever," p. 681.

35. For a discussion of the theological perception of cholera, 1832–1866, see Charles E. Rosenberg, *The Cholera Years: The United States in 1832, 1849, and 1866* (Chicago: University of Chicago Press, 1962). See also Shryock, *Medicine and Society*, p. 94; *Rush Letters*, 2: 659; Horace W. Smith, *Life and Correspondence of the Rev. William Smith, D.D.,* . . . 2 vols. (Philadelphia: Ferguson Brothers, 1880), 1: 395; *General Advertiser*, 8 January 1794.

36. Rush to William Marshall, 15 September 1798, in *Rush Letters*, 2: 807. Rush also blamed party spirit in general. See also *National Gazette*, 9, 12, and 16 October 1793; Carey, *Short Account*, p. 10.

37. Smith, *Life of William Smith*, 1: 392.

38. Graydon, *Memoirs*, p. 335; Stephen G. Kurtz, *The Presidency of John Adams: The Collapse of Federalism, 1795–1800* (Philadelphia: University of Pennsylvania Press, 1957), p. 190; Charles D. Hazen, *Contemporary American Opinion of the French Revolution* (Baltimore: Johns Hopkins University Press, 1897), pp. 185–186.

39. *National Gazette*, 16 October 1793; Scharf and Westcott, *Philadelphia*, 2: 966–967.

40. Ibid.

41. *Gazette of the United States*, 19, 28 December 1793; *General Advertiser*, 6 January 1794; Arthur Hornblow, *History of the Theatre in America*, 2 vols. (Philadelphia and London: J.B. Lippincott Co., 1919), 1: 174–175; *National Gazette*, 16 October 1793.

42. *Gazette of the United States,* 14, 26 December 1793, 8 February 1794; René La Roche, *Yellow Fever Considered in Its Historical, Pathological, Etiological, and Therapeutical Relations . . .* (Philadelphia: Blanchard and Lea, 1855), p. 73; William Priest, *Travels in the United States of America . . .* (London: Printed for J. Johnson, 1802), p. 13; [John Purdon], *A Leisure Hour; or a Series of Poetical Letters, Mostly Written During the Prevalence of the Yellow Fever* (Philadelphia: Printed and Sold by P. Stewart, 1804), p. 27.
43. Several leading Republican literary figures remained aloof from this alliance. Bache, whose son-in-law was an actor, was accused of misrepresenting rank-and-file Republican sentiment on the theater for family reasons. Rufus Griswold, *The Republican Court; or, American Society in the Days of Washington* (New York: Appleton, 1854), p. 316; *General Advertiser,* 10 January 1794. On 8 January, though, Bache attributed his stand to anticlericalism. See also Mathew Carey, *Autobiography* (1837; reprint, New York: E.L. Schwab, 1942), p. 29.
44. W. H. Hargreaves and R. J. G. Morrison, *The Practice of Tropical Medicine* (London: Staples, 1965), pp. 183–185; Powell, *Bring Out Your Dead,* pp. 64, 125, 292. Wine is generally not a stimulant although it was believed to be one. Chris Holmes, "Benjamin Rush and the Yellow Fever," *Bulletin of the History of Medicine* 40 (1966): 246–262, believes Rush's cures were not lethal, but does not fully distinguish patients like Hazard, who left Rush after one or two treatments, from those who stayed for the full course of bloodletting.
45. David Freeman Hawke, *Benjamin Rush, Revolutionary Gadfly* (Indianapolis: Bobbs-Merrill, 1971), pp. 208–223, 236–240; Powell, *Bring Out Your Dead,* p. 78; Goodman, *Benjamin Rush,* pp. 90–116.
46. Powell, *Bring Out Your Dead,* pp. 82, 153, 203; George Logan to "Citizen Bache," in *General Advertiser,* 18 September 1793; *The Papers of Alexander Hamilton,* ed. Harold C. Syrett and Jacob E. Cooke, 27 vols. (New York: Columbia University Press, 1961–1987), 15: 325 n. 1. Say's party affiliation is derived from Tinkcom, *Republicans and Federalists,* p. 240.
47. *Dunlap's American Daily Advertiser,* 13 September 1793; *Hamilton Papers,* 15: 331–332; Powell, *Bring Out Your Dead,* p. 135; Goodman, *Benjamin Rush,* p. 215; Jenkins, *Washington in Germantown,* p. 25.
48. B. Rush to J. Rush, 3 October 1793, to Horatio Gates, 26 December 1795, to John Dickinson, 11 October 1797, in *Rush Letters,* 2: 701, 767, 793; Goodman, *Benjamin Rush,* pp. 203, 209.
49. McFarland, "Yellow Fever and Dr. Rush," pp. 486–487; John E. Lane, "Jean Devèze," *Annals of Medical History,* n.s., 8 (1936): 220; Margaret Woodbury, *Public Opinion in Philadelphia, 1789–1801* (Northampton, Mass.: Department of History of Smith College, 1920), p. 16; and Goodman, *Benjamin Rush,* p. 208. Some Republican bark physicians agreed that Rush's cures were egalitarian but denied that political Republicanism required opposition to medical elitism. See letter of "Citizen Robert, M.D.," *General Advertiser,* 6 December 1793, whose combination of titles reflects his attempt to combine egalitarianism and professional distinctions.
50. Powell, *Bring Out Your Dead,* p. 201; *Rush Letters,* 2: 692.

51. McFarland, "Yellow Fever and Dr. Rush," p. 462.

52. Goodman, *Benjamin Rush*, p. 183.

53. Stephen Girard to Pierre Changeur & Co., 11 September 1793, Girard Papers, American Philosophical Society; Powell, *Bring Out Your Dead*, pp. 175, 179–180.

54. Powell, *Bring Out Your Dead*, pp. 179, 242. Samuel Coates is not to be confused with William Coates, a founder of the Democratic Society. Henry Simpson, *The Lives of Eminent Philadelphians, Now Deceased* (Philadelphia: W. Brotherhead, 1859), p. 218; *Gazette of the United States*, 14 December 1793.

55. Carey, *Short Account*, pp. 27, 28. Carey seems to slight Federalists in his stories of heroism. For their side, see also *Extracts from the Diary of Jacob Hiltzheimer, of Philadelphia*, ed. Jacob Cox Parsons (Philadelphia: Press of W.F. Fell and Co., 1893), pp. 195–197; Smith, *Life of William Smith*, 1: 379; Upham, *Life of Pickering*, 3: 62; "Hazard Letters," p. 334; Powell, *Bring Out Your Dead*, p. 138; and Simpson, *Eminent Philadelphians*, pp. 908–922. For party affiliations of Morris (as of 1798), see letter of 19 November 1798, Hollingsworth MSS; of Humphreys, see Scharf and Westcott, *Philadelphia*, 1: 490; of Hollingsworth, see David Hackett Fischer, *The Revolution of American Conservatism: The Federalist Party in the Era of Jeffersonian Democracy* (New York: Harper and Row, 1965), p. 339; of Hiltzheimer and FitzSimmons, see Tinkcom, *Republicans and Federalists*, pp. 138, 152. In addition, Samuel Pancoast of the merchants' committee was listed as a Federalist by 1817. Scharf and Westcott, *Philadelphia*, 1: 588.

56. For Wetherill, see Simpson, *Eminent Philadelphians*, p. 940, and Tinkcom, *Republicans and Federalists*, p. 252; for Lownes, see Scharf and Westcott, *Philadelphia*, 1: 477; for Girard, see Link, *Democratic Societies*, pp. 75–76; for Israel, see Powell, *Bring Out Your Dead*, p. 178; for Carey, see Carey, *Autobiography*; for Sergeant, see *Dictionary of American Biography*, s.v. "Sergeant, Jonathan Dickinson"; for Sharswood, see Simpson, *Eminent Philadelphians*, p. 885; for Kerr and Connelly, see Minute Book of the Democratic Society, pp. 29, 47, Historical Society of Pennsylvania, and Scharf and Westcott, *Philadelphia*, 1: 507, 588; for Wistar, see Powell, *Bring Out Your Dead*, p. 179. The list of leaders of the committee was compiled from names most frequently cited in *Minutes of the Proceedings of the Committee Appointed on the 14th September, 1793* (Philadelphia: Printed by R. Aitken and Son, 1848); and Carey, *Short Account*, p. 95.

57. Powell, *Bring Out Your Dead*, pp. 72, 87, 179; Ford, *David Rittenhouse*, p. 190; and Kenneth R. Rossman, *Thomas Mifflin and the Politics of the American Revolution* (Chapel Hill: University of North Carolina Press, 1952), p. 225.

58. Powell, *Bring Out Your Dead*, p. 177; and Ford, *David Rittenhouse*, pp. 190–192.

59. Helm was Girard's assistant in charge of "external affairs." He was a second generation German-American but little else is known of him. The chronology of Bush Hill is as follows: 31 August—Mayor authorizes seizure of estate, hospital set up under Leib and others; 16 September—Girard and Helm volunteer to manage and administer the hospital for the committee; 18 September—Girard appoints Devèze to assist Leib and the medical staff; 21 September—Leib resigns in dispute over the proper cure. Powell, *Bring Out Your Dead*, pp. 140–172.

60. Democratic Society Minute Book, pp. 29, 39, 42, 47, 48, 52, 95; Link, *Democratic Societies*, 77, 90; Carey, *Short Account*, pp. 20, 27, 30, 37; Tinkcom, *Republicans and*

Federalists, pp. 57, 84, 283. Snyder is identified as of 1799 in Scharf and Westcott, *Philadelphia*, 1: 507, 588. There were two John Barclays; this one was president of the Republican Bank of Pennsylvania. Duplication of names makes it impossible to say whether merchants' committeeman William Clifton was the Federalist poet or one of two shopkeepers of that name. Likewise, William Sansom, Guardian of the Poor, may have been either the Federalist or the Republican of that name. Simpson, *Eminent Philadelphians*, p. 210; General Roll of McPherson's Blues, Hollingsworth MSS; J. Hardie, *The Philadelphia Directory and Register* . . . (Philadelphia: Printed for the Author by T. Dobson, 1793), p. 182 and passim.

61. Powell, *Bring Out Your Dead*, pp. 85–86. To avoid confusion over the new implications of its old name, the *Federal Gazette* became the *Philadelphia Gazette* on 1 January 1794. Clarence S. Brigham, *History and Bibliography of American Newspapers, 1690–1820*, 2 vols. (Worcester, Mass.: American Antiquarian Society, 1947), 2: 91.

62. Lewis Leary, *That Rascal Freneau: A Study in Literary Failure* (New Brunswick, N.J.: Rutgers University Press, 1941), pp. 240–246; Dumas Malone, *Jefferson and the Ordeal of Liberty*, Vol. 3 of *Jefferson and His Time* 6 vols. (Boston: Little, Brown, 1962), 3: 142.

63. *National Gazette*, 11 September 1793, 9 October 1793; Scharf and Westcott, *Philadelphia*, 2: 1606; *Minutes of the Committee*, p. 232.

64. Powell's account, *Bring Out Your Dead*, p. 135, differs from Rush's version of the Van Berkle business, B. Rush to J. Rush, 3 October 1793, in *Rush Letters*, 2: 701. Wolcott fled with Knox in early September. Jenkins, *Washington in Germantown*, p. 22.

65. Powell, *Bring Out Your Dead*, p. 123.

66. Jefferson to Madison, 8 September 1793, in *The Writings of Thomas Jefferson*, ed. Paul Leicester Ford, 10 vols. (New York: G.P. Putnam's Sons, 1895), 6: 419; Malone, *Jefferson and the Ordeal of Liberty*, pp. 140–142.

67. *National Gazette*, 4 September 1793. The version in Powell, *Bring Out Your Dead*, p. 240, is not the original 1793 poem but a printed edition of 1795. The original attacks all deserters; the later one absolves all but the fleeing physicians. Condemnation of the fugitives often stressed their wealth. *Gazette of the United States*, letter of 20 February 1794.

68. *Dunlap's American Daily Advertiser*, 14 December 1793; Nathaniel Burt, *The Perennial Philadelphians: The Anatomy of an American Aristocracy* (Boston: Little, Brown, 1963), pp. 156–157. "Nomination," "platform," etc. are all useful metaphors in spite of the anachronism.

69. *Gazette of the United States*, 13 December 1793.

70. Ibid., 14, 20 December 1793; Robert C. Alberts, *The Golden Voyage: The Life and Times of William Bingham, 1752–1804* (Boston: Houghton Mifflin, 1969), p. 246. Out of 14,000 eligible, only 1,282 Philadelphians came out to vote. *Independent Gazetteer*, 21 December 1793.

71. *Dunlap's American Daily Advertiser*, 14 December 1793.

72. *Hamilton Papers*, 15: 332 n; Carey, *Short Account*, p. 93; Powell, *Bring Out Your Dead*, pp. 216–232.

73. *General Advertiser*, 2 December 1793; *Rush Letters*, 2: 736; Johnson, *Account*, p. 28; Powell, *Bring Out Your Dead*, pp. 87, 178. Carey printed rumors of black profiteering similar to Johnson's but he hastily withdrew them. Richard Allen, *Life Experi-*

ences and Gospel Labors (Philadelphia: Martin and Boden, Printers, 1933), pp. 34–35.

74. *General Advertiser*, 2, 3 December 1793; *Federal Gazette*, 9, 14 December 1793.

75. "HOWARD," in *General Advertiser*, 8 January 1794; see also 27 November 1793.

76. Tinkcom, *Republicans and Federalists*, pp. 176–179; John Bach McMaster, *The Life and Times of Stephen Girard, Mariner and Merchant*, 2 vols. (Philadelphia: Lippincott, 1918), 1: 352. The career of Israel Israel and his role in Philadelphia class politics is traced in John K. Alexander, "The City of Brotherly Fear: The Poor in Late-Eighteenth-Century Philadelphia," in Kenneth T. Jackson and Stanley K. Schultz, comps., *Cities in American History* (New York: Knopf, 1972), pp. 86–90.

77. *The Works of John Adams . . .*, ed. Charles Francis Adams, 10 vols. (Boston: Little, Brown, 1856), 10: 47. Jefferson declared the death of Hutchinson to be as great a setback as the Genêt fiasco. Merrill D. Peterson, *Thomas Jefferson and the New Nation: A Biography* (New York: Oxford University Press, 1970), p. 508.

78. Tinkcom, *Republicans and Federalists*, p. 173.

79. Jean Pierre Blanchard had recently introduced the city to the French hot air balloon.

80. Two of Rush's black apprentices.

81. *Gazette of the United States*, 23 December 1793.

Afterword

82. Kenneth Kiple and Virginia Kiple, "Black Yellow Fever Immunities, Innate and Acquired, as Revealed in the American South," *Social Science History* 1 (1977): 419–36. Also see K. David Patterson, "Yellow Fever Epidemics and Mortality in the U.S., 1693–1905," *Social Science and Medicine* 34 (1992): 855–65.

83. For example, Margaret Pelling, *Cholera, Fever, and English Medicine* (New York: Oxford University Press, 1978); Dale C. Smith, ed., *William Budd On the Causes of Fevers (1839)* (Baltimore: Johns Hopkins University Press, 1984); and Margaret DeLacy, "The Conceptualization of Influenza in Eighteenth-Century Britain: Specificity and Contagion," *Bulletin of the History of Medicine* 67 (Spring 1993): 74–118.

84. For example, Eve Kornfeld asserted that the paper overemphasizes the role of politics in what she believes was essentially a cultural debate. But I concluded that Rush and Hamilton *failed* in their effort to politicize physicians' actual choices of therapy, and that the Republicans *failed* in their efforts to gain politically from their heroism. I was trying to show the interconnection of politics and culture (and medicine), not to reduce one to the other. Eve Kornfeld, "Crisis in the Capital: Cultural Significance of Philadelphia's Great Yellow Fever Epidemic," *Pennsylvania History* 51 (1984): 189–205.

Comment: Disease
and Community

BILLY G. SMITH

HEY are a Dieing on our right hand & on our Left, we have it oposit us, in fact, all around us, great are the number that are Calld to the grave. . . . [T]o se[e] the hurst [hearse] go by, is now so common, that we hardly take notice of it, in fine we live in the midst of Death." So wrote Philadelphian Isaac Heston to his brother on 19 September 1793 at a time when yellow fever claimed the lives of about 70 of the city's residents each day. "When I se[e] the Metropolis of the United States depopulated," the twenty-two-year-old moaned, "it is too distressing and afecting a sean, for a person young in Life to bear." Heston died ten days later from the disease.[1]

Heston's poignant personal testimony of despair resonates with us two hundred years later in part because his tragic circumstances are all too familiar in the 1990s. The twentieth century has been filled with death and destruction. From trench warfare in World War I and the deadly worldwide influenza after the conflagration, to the Holocaust and nuclear weapons in World War II, to genocide in Cambodia, Bosnia, and Rwanda, to the recent reappearance of plague in India and famine in Ethiopia, people living in the twentieth century have suffered the horrors of numerous catastrophes created both by human hands and by "natural disasters" like disease, floods, and famines.

Recently, as the Cold War ended and the potential of vast nuclear destruction abated, the dangers of disease-causing microbes throughout the planet intensified. AIDS, resulting from the human immunodeficiency virus (HIV), is now a world-wide phenomenon, while other new viruses like Ebola and Marburg exact a price for modern material "progress" as people encroach on jungles and rain forests and otherwise disrupt numerous local habitats. Meanwhile, well-known bacterial species are evolving strains resistant to antibiotics, so that previously "controllable" diseases like tuberculosis and polio pose renewed threats to human health. Familiar maladies like yellow fever continue their relentless destruction of thousands of lives, especially in the world's poorer tropical areas. Lamentably, humans have used modern medicine to eradicate only a handful of diseases, smallpox being the most notable.[2]

Disease, of course, has played a critical role in human history, especially since Europe began its global expansion five centuries ago. Smallpox and measles were two of the biological bullets in the arsenal of Europeans which helped them conquer Native Americans. Malaria, yellow fever, and other maladies shielded some tropical regions of Africa and Asia from European invasion until the advent of tropical medicines like quinine. More recently, AIDS and other sexually transmitted diseases have altered the nature of intimacy and gender relations throughout the world. HIV and other new viruses pose special threats to the peoples of Africa, threatening to depopulate that continent during the coming decades, much as many of the natives of America were destroyed after the arrival of Europeans.[3]

This new, global epidemiological dilemma provides a context for reconsidering an epidemic in the nation's capital two hundred years ago. The essays in this volume analyze how Philadelphians responded to the 1793 yellow fever epidemic, attributed meaning to that event, fashioned medical theories and treatments about the disease, and proposed and implemented preventive measures for the future. This analysis helps us comprehend a great deal about the social, political, and economic concerns of citizens in the new nation, and how those concerns shaped the ways in which Americans interpreted the viral attack and conducted themselves during the crisis. A more thorough understanding of these issues may enable us to probe more deeply into questions about how and why humankind is reacting (or failing to react) to the current peril posed by diverse diseases.

This "Comment" is divided into two parts. First, it will highlight some of the basic features of the epidemic, many of which are considered but a few of which are ignored in this volume. These issues include the history and origins of yellow fever in Philadelphia, the transmission of the disease, the special vulnerability of particular residents to its attack, the problems encountered by survivors of the epidemic, and the place of yellow fever in the city's epidemiological environment. Second, the arguments of the essays in this volume will be evaluated as they relate to both ideas and reality about the "communities" which constituted Philadelphia in the 1790s.

Yellow fever periodically devastated Philadelphia after its founding in 1682. The worst incident occurred in 1699 when a third of the white residents and an unknown number of slaves died. The disease appeared at least five more times during the colonial period, driving the death rates to extraordinary heights in 1741 and 1762. After an absence of more than three decades, yellow fever again struck the city in 1793, tripling the annual crude death rates of the preceding five years. According to Susan E. Klepp's careful assessment of the best available evidence, death rates among Philadelphia's original inhabitants averaged between 64 and 98 per thousand of those infected during that epidemic (although not all deaths resulted directly from yellow fever). Among residents who did not flee the city, fatality was considerably higher: as many as one of every five of them died. Yellow fever reappeared in Philadelphia and attacked other northern American urban centers intermittently during the summers and falls for at least the next dozen years, although the death toll gradually lessened as many survivors acquired immunity from having contracted the disease previously.[4]

Just as the increased movement of people and goods during the past few decades has spread disease on a global scale, migration and commerce in the eighteenth-century Atlantic World bore similar ghastly consequences. Philadelphians engaged in brisk trade with the West Indies throughout the century, and ships arriving from the Caribbean probably introduced the *Aedes aegypti*, one of the few species of mosquitoes capable of carrying yellow fever, as well as the infected passengers on whom the insects fed. A viral disease common to the tropics and initially conveyed to America from Africa, yellow fever is transmitted from one infected person (or monkey) to another through the sting of the *Aedes aegypti*. The virus invades the liver and produces a yellow color in its host as liver function fails, thereby giving the disease its name. Mosquitoes aboard vessels docking in Philadelphia found a hospitable environment in the marshes west of the city and in Dock Creek, a stream which barely oozed from the swamps through the city's heart to the Delaware River. The *Aedes aegypti* is well adapted to urban conditions since it thrives, according to Klepp, in "small, calm bodies of water . . . such as the water barrels on board ships, the rain barrels Philadelphians left next to their houses, or even an undisturbed wash basin or forgotten glass of water." The mosquito's limited range, Klepp notes, meant that yellow fever "rarely appeared far from the waterfront and almost never in the countryside." Similar to other diseases spread by insects, yellow fever occurred seasonally, usually beginning in late July or August, peaking in September and October, then ending quickly in November as cold weather froze or otherwise incapacitated the harbingers of death.[5]

Given the state of medical knowledge, Philadelphia's physicians, as J. Worth Estes explains, could do nothing to halt the disease. Yet they tried valiantly, proposing a host of theories and therapies. Ordinary citizens often distrusted and were confused by the contradictory treatments recommended by doctors, and they resorted to additional measures to protect themselves. They fired muskets, chewed garlic, burned bonfires, rang bells, smoked their bedding and houses with tobacco, and carried pieces of tarred rope, all, of course, to no avail.[6]

The only sure means to avoid the disease was to escape the city entirely, as Benjamin Rush advised. Philadelphia's wealthiest citizens traditionally moved to their country estates to avoid the dreaded "summer complaints" and the "fall agues" which regularly afflicted the city during warmer months. But in 1793, residents departed in record number. As Alexander Graydon reported, "Those whose property enabled them to do it fled with precipitation." Between a third and a half of the inhabitants beat a hasty retreat. "So great was the general terror," Mathew Carey remarked, "that for some weeks, carts, waggons, coaches, and [riding] chairs, were almost constantly transporting families and furniture to the country in every direction." Social and economic life in the Quaker City halted abruptly as people "shut themselves up in their houses, and were afraid to walk the streets." Sea captains refused to dock their ships and farmers declined to transport their produce into the city. "Business," Carey declared, "then became extremely dull." Residents who remained in the city, even if they did not contract the fever, consequently suffered from unemployment, poverty, and, in some cases, deprivation of the necessities of life. Meanwhile, death carts rumbled through the streets constantly; the wagons picked up more than five hundred bodies in a single five-day period in October.[7]

Yellow fever killed Philadelphians selectively, in part reflecting crucial differences among the city's inhabitants. The epidemic, as Klepp notes, was particularly grave for "young and middle-aged adults, the poor, men and native-born or European-born whites." Once afflicted, children and infants survived in greater numbers because, as is the general pattern, they experienced milder cases of the disease than did adults. Women fared better than men, perhaps because women fled more quickly or were sent out of the city by their husbands and fathers. Because many were migrants who had contracted yellow fever and thereby gained immunity to the microbes in the South, Africa, or the West Indies, black Philadelphians experienced lower death rates than whites. For the same reason, the French residents in the city who had fled the slave revolution in the Caribbean apparently suffered relatively few fatalities.

The yellow fever virus was also class specific, taking an especially heavy toll among Philadelphia's "lower sort" (as they were labeled by contemporaries). The disease was "dreadfully destructive among the poor," Carey noted. "It is very probable that at least seven eighths of the number of the dead, was of that class." His observation is confirmed by the disproportionate number of mariners, laborers, artisans, clothes washers, and prostitutes among the victims.[8] Inferior diets, overcrowded housing, and inadequate sanitary conditions intensified the vulnerability of the lower classes to yellow fever. Most important was the inability of impoverished residents to escape the afflicted area. As one newspaper essayist recognized during a subsequent epidemic, departing the city was impossible for "the poor who have neither places to remove to or funds for their support, as they depend on their daily labour, for daily supplies."[9] The small red flags that, by order of the Board of Health, adorned the doors of houses containing people infected by the fever proliferated in the alleys and lanes occupied by poorer Philadelphians in the city's center. Nearly a third of the residents of Moravian Alley, for example, and a half of those in Fetter Lane succumbed to the disease in 1793. Jacob Flake, a tailor living at the end of Moravian Alley, lost six children to the pestilence; "whole families," according to Carey, sank "into one silent, undistinguished grave."[10]

While the many lives ended prematurely by yellow fever were the most tragic aspect of the epidemic, survivors also suffered extreme emotional and financial distress. Jacob Flake and his wife must have found it nearly unbearable to cope with the death of their six children. Women widowed by the epidemic often were forced to struggle hard to make ends meet, especially if they had children to support. After Susannah Cook lost both her husband, a successful hairdresser, and a son during the epidemic, she washed clothes and took in boarders to maintain herself and two surviving children. The laborious work may have contributed to the destruction of her own health, since she died in the almshouse eight years later. The disease also orphaned scores of children, many of whom were apprenticed by the Guardians of the Poor.[11]

Even though the 1793 epidemic is the one in early America best remembered by subsequent generations, Klepp reminds us that it was neither the most fatal epidemic in an American city, nor was it as lethal as some other diseases. Yellow fever claimed the lives of a greater proportion of Philadelphia's inhabitants in 1699 than in 1793. And throughout the colonial era, smallpox was more deadly on a continual basis, although its virulence declined during the century's final three decades as variolation—an early form of vaccination—increased. Although yellow fever reappeared four times in the city during the 1790s, tuberculosis (then known as "consumption") accounted for even more deaths. Measles, diphtheria, whooping cough, and various enigmatic "fevers" likewise terminated many lives, while convulsions and diarrhea were especially fatal to infants.[12]

The excellent studies in this volume use the 1793 epidemic both as a window through which to view life in the early nation and as a means to comment on issues relevant to the present day. One theme that pervades the essays and which is pertinent to America in the 1990s concerns the nature of the "community" or "communities" which constituted Philadelphia. How were these communities defined? Who was included and who was excluded? How did the official community disintegrate during the epidemic and by what means was it reconstructed? How did the political perspective of the community affect proposed medical treatments? What type of community did people hope or fear would develop in the new nation? How did Philadelphians act as a community after the epidemics to improve the city? The remainder of my comment focuses on the ways in which the authors address these questions.

David Paul Nord is intrigued primarily by the civic function of newspapers. He adroitly uses the 1793 crisis as a microscope through which to observe the readers of the *Federal Gazette*—the only newspaper that published throughout the epidemic—and to scrutinize the reasons why they both read and wrote to the newspaper. Philadelphians turned to the *Gazette* as a source of "authentic intelligence" about what was happening in their city, although they (like many readers today) often were frustrated to find rumors, confusion, and medical debates (parallel to today's confusing arguments about health care, the causes of cancer, and AIDS) instead of accurate information. In the midst of a terrifying catastrophe, Philadelphians also wrote to the newspaper to share their personal experiences, suggest cures for the disease, advise city officials about the proper measures to adopt, offer religious interpretations of the pestilence, and even proffer bleak satires of the tragic event. By these actions, Philadelphians not only endorsed the Revolutionary ideology of the equality of ideas of all people but also participated in creating a community of citizens.

Although Nord provides an excellent analysis of the ways in which Philadelphia's newspapers helped construct "new forms of public community in the modern, impersonal metropolis," he is perhaps overly enthusiastic about the importance of the print medium. Eventually he succumbs to the "self-congratulatory rhetoric" that he accuses newspaper editors of too easily embracing, and he exaggerates the significance of newspapers. The *Federal Gazette* not only maintained a sense of community, Nord contends, but communication itself became "the fundamental bond of society." Yet, could newspapers have played such a significant role in a city where so many people were illiterate and where nearly everyone was afraid during the epidemic to venture outside their homes?

During the 1790s, Philadelphia was the country's primary immigrant port of entry, and many of the migrants who washed into the city remained permanently beached there. The result was an urban center marked by remarkable ethnic and racial variety, swimming with natives from northern Europe, Great Britain, the West Indies, Africa, and rural areas of North America. Many in this tide of new arrivals could neither read nor speak English, and few could afford to buy newspapers on a regular basis. Reports in the *Federal Gazette* about the course and possible cure of yellow fever would have been of interest to immigrants and others among the lower classes, but the newspaper would not necessarily have provided them with a sense of belonging to a unified community. Indeed, a substantial number of Philadelphians of all classes did not attend a church, or send their children to a school, or vote in local elections, or reside near relatives, or live in stable neighborhoods. Rather than belonging to a community, they experienced, suffered, and sometimes undoubtedly even enjoyed the anonymity of urban life.[13]

Religion and economics probably played more substantial roles than communication in shaping people's definition of their community and in holding society together. Surely the religious concerns of Philadelphians immersed daily in life and death struggles must have intensified greatly during the pestilential siege. In a diary written during a less severe yellow fever epidemic in 1798, Benjamin Garrigues, overwhelmed by fears about his own mortality, invoked God's protection on a daily and sometimes even hourly basis. Simultaneously, Garrigues ministered to the sick, partly out of a sense of religious duty, and regularly attended worship services. This dedication both to religious ideals and to helping other people may well have bound some Philadelphians tightly together, at least for the duration of the epidemic. In addition, financial problems, exacerbated when the economy stopped functioning during the crisis, became an issue for nearly everyone left in the city. Officials responded by borrowing thousands of dollars to purchase and distribute food and other necessities, while dozens of ministers preached "charity sermons" to raise funds for the poor. Such actions seemingly were more important than a single newspaper in strengthening communal bonds among Philadelphians.[14]

As Nord clearly recognizes, Philadelphia's newspapers did not produce a single city-wide community, although they did contribute to the creation of a fellowship among more affluent citizens. Eighteenth-century Philadelphia was characterized by deep social and economic fissures. The city was comprised of a multitude of communities, many of them defined and separated by race, class, gender, and ethnicity. Nord indicates that it is highly unlikely that each of these groups of citizens read the *Federal Gazette* during the epidemic and discovered there a shared sense of commonality with other like-minded citizens. Instead, the "middling" and "better sort" (as they were called at the time) likely constituted the primary audience for Philadelphia's newspapers since those publications specialized in providing information valuable to their interests. Advertisements for slaves, servants, horses, and cows; notices of the sale of real estate and merchandise; and listings of ship arrivals and departures as well as the current prices of goods at home and abroad filled most of the space in eighteenth-century newspapers. Husbands also occasionally advertised for runaway wives to prevent shopkeepers from extending them credit, while masters offered rewards for escaped servants and slaves.

While the news media undoubtedly helped create a sense of community in Philadelphia before, during, and after the epidemic, it was one comprised overwhelmingly of prosperous white males. This was not a fellowship which bound *all* Philadelphians together since some benefited while others suffered from the information disseminated by the newspapers. As Nord observes, newspapers "have often been instruments of division as well as connection," and in this case poorer white males, unfree people, and women were largely excluded from the community of readers.

African Americans, who accounted for approximately one of every ten Philadelphians during the 1790s, did not belong to the community defined by newspaper readers. Not only were the great majority of blacks illiterate, but the numerous advertisements in the *Federal Gazette* and other city newspapers offering bondpeople for sale or rewards for runaway slaves were unlikely to have won the hearts and minds of black Philadelphians. For African Americans, the print medium operated more as an organ of oppression than as an instrument of unity.

Phillip Lapsansky skillfully documents how black Philadelphians actively assisted their white neighbors during the epidemic by attending the sick and burying the dead. As Isaac Heston noted in the midst of the suffering, "I dont know what the people would do, if it was not for the Negroes, as they are the Principal nurses."[15] During the crisis, according to Lapsansky, blacks "helped administer what was effectively the government of the city," perhaps the first time in the history of an American metropolis that its black citizenry wielded such authority. Although many African Americans perished, a handful of unfree blacks (and bound white servants) actually benefited from the epidemics. Some slaves and servants took advantage of the chaos created by the pestilence to escape, while others gained their liberty when their masters died.

Frequently in the American past, whites have expected blacks to "prove" themselves worthy of citizenship by making sacrifices during wars, natural disasters, and other crisis events. African Americans have often responded, in part because of their commitment to a larger multiracial community, in part for their own immediate benefit, and in part as an attempt to force whites to recognize their status as equal partners in American society. During the 1793 epidemic, black Philadelphians laid their lives on the line for all of these reasons. But when Mathew Carey publicly derided the actions of African Americans during the epidemic, "what hope was there," Lapsansky asks, "for the wider acceptance of blacks as freemen and citizens?" Outraged, Richard Allen and Absalom Jones responded by writing "the first account of a free black community in action," and "the first African American polemic in which black leaders sought to articulate black community anger and directly confront an accuser." As a result, Carey softened his criticism of blacks in subsequent editions of his account of the epidemic. The laudable behavior of African Americans also may have helped soften the racial attitudes of many white Philadelphians, if only briefly during the 1790s, as Gary B. Nash found in his study of race relations in Philadelphia.[16] Still, regardless of the participation of blacks in saving Philadelphia during the epidemic, whites ultimately refused to embrace them as either citizens or equals.

Ironically, African Americans, although the most despised group in the city merely because of their race, were among the Philadelphians most successful in forging their own community during the late eighteenth century. As a large number of free blacks and escaped slaves congregated in an American metropolis for the first time, they lived and worked together to establish churches, schools, and other institutions which defined their community.[17]

Sally F. Griffith's impressive analysis of Mathew Carey's chronicle of the epidemic reminds us that "instant histories" are not solely the preserve of late-twentieth-century journalists. Griffith interprets this well-known account as a narrative of the death and rebirth of a community. From Carey's perspective of providential republicanism, Philadelphians had fallen from grace by abandoning the central Revolutionary ideals of virtue and sobriety in favor of luxury and extravagance in the years preceding the epidemic. The community thus was ripe for collapse when afflicted by pestilence. Ultimately the disease, in Griffith's eloquent words, induced "a sort of social hell, a reversion to a brutal, Hobbesian state of nature." Only the heroic, selfless actions of a small group of people, claims Carey, created a new social compact, regenerated essential institutions, and saved the city. But if Carey recounts an inspiring story of the heroism of white males, he fails, Griffith observes, to credit the significant contributions made by other Philadelphians. In particular, Carey takes little note of women and, as Lapsansky discusses, he denigrates the conduct of African Americans, even though both groups were critical in nursing the city back to health.

At the conclusion of her essay, Griffith speculates that Carey's "narrative of community destruction and regeneration has continued to influence the ways Americans have responded to . . . civic disasters." Griffith's efforts to link the past and the present are intriguing and commendable. But do Americans who experience community-wide devastation really look to the past— and specifically to the yellow fever epidemics—to determine their behavior or their understanding of the event? Few Americans today have any knowledge of the epidemics of the 1790s or of Carey's account. Moreover, if the yellow fever epidemics had never occurred or if Carey had never written his account, it still seems likely that citizen committees would have formed and volunteers would have appeared to offer assistance to the victims of the 1993 floods in the Mississippi River Valley.

The ways in which Americans approach and interpret tragic events which destroy their communities have changed significantly over the past two centuries, particularly during the last 50 years. While Americans still expect that citizen volunteers will play a leading role in reconstructing their towns and cities, they also presume that the federal and state governments in conjunction with private insurance companies will assume the primary responsibility for repairing the damage inflicted by floods, hurricanes, or even plagues of frogs, and for physically reconstructing their communities. Moreover, relatively few Americans, except for some fundamentalist Christians, now believe that natural disasters are part of God's retribution for the nation having fallen from grace or sacrificed its soul to materialism. The jeremiad narrative tradition to which Carey's account belongs resonates considerably less with Americans in the late twentieth century than it did previously.

Still, two notable events, one recent and another contemporaneous with the 1793 epidemic, resemble Carey's chronicle in some respects and support Griffith's hypothesis. First, a striking modern parallel to Carey's account has been the initial devastation of the homosexual community by AIDS (although the disease, of course, attacks heterosexuals as well). Subsequently, however, gays and lesbians have reconstructed their communities by engaging in a remarkable struggle against both a hideous disease and hideously biased attitudes which suffuse American society. Unfortunately, some religious conservatives mirror Carey's notion when they proclaim that the disease is God's scourge sent to punish homosexuals for their supposed transgression of Biblical morality.

Second, a few hundred miles to the north of Philadelphia, the Seneca, a tribal group belonging to the Iroquois Confederacy, suffered incredible demographic, economic, political, and cultural decimation in the aftermath of the American Revolution. At the same time that Philadelphians were rebuilding their institutions, a visionary named Handsome Lake helped the Seneca to revivify and redefine their society by combining elements of both Native American and European cultures. Ironically, in both of these instances, the death and rebirth of communities involved people who traditionally have been excluded from full membership in American society.[18]

Jacquelyn C. Miller retells the familiar story of Benjamin Rush and his controversial treatment of yellow fever during the 1793 epidemic, but she recasts it in a new form. Miller's remarkable essay examines the connection between Rush's proposed radical treatment of the disease and his political beliefs, especially those centering around his vision of the nature of the community which he hoped would define the new nation. Rush's "reaction to the epidemic is best understood within the context of his larger social and political concerns," Miller argues, and "his response should be envisioned as a struggle to avert a second American Revolution." Like Martin S. Pernick's path-breaking study undertaken twenty years ago (and reprinted in this volume), Miller's analysis reminds us that medicine, like all science, is not totally objective but instead often is influenced by social and political concerns. Thus, the convictions of many of the city's medical men about the origins and, occasionally, even the proper treatment of the disease were shaped partly by their own political perspectives.

Like most of the famous founding fathers, including John Adams, James Madison, and George Washington, Benjamin Rush embraced the republican notion that government should rest on the consent of the governed, yet he doubted the ability of the mass of humanity to govern themselves. Poor white males posed the greatest threat to the existence of the new American nation since they were beginning to flex their political muscle, yet they were ruled too often by their passions and they would pursue policies which would benefit their class rather than the country as a whole. According to this intellectual formulation, only people who owned property and therefore had a stake in society and the social order were capable of acting rationally, objectively, and in a virtuous manner productive of the "common good." The American Revolution unleashed dangerous democratic tendencies, Rush feared, as evidenced in the significant extension of the franchise by the Pennsylvania Constitution of 1776. The excesses of the French Revolution frightened conservative American leaders even more. For the new American nation to succeed, order must be restored, democracy must be restrained, and the passions of the lower sort must be contained.

Rush believed that the health of the community and the health of the human body were intimately intertwined. He assumed, according to Miller, "that the organization of social and political systems and the health of the people who populated those systems were so mutually related that any widespread modifications in social relationships produced accompanying changes in the health of the peoples involved." When Rush proposed excessive purging and bleeding of up to 80 percent of the blood in the bodies of patients, he was responding not only to the yellow fever catastrophe but also to the political crisis caused by excessive democracy. Bleeding was a way to control the passions of both the physical body and the body politic, and particularly of the lower classes. Many of the patients whom Rush treated during the epidemic, it should be added, undoubtedly belonged to the lower sort, since they were the ones who lacked the financial wherewithal to flee the city. Rush was literally draining poorer people of their blood, their passions, and, sometimes, their lives. (Rush's radical prescription, William Cobbett commented wryly, was "one of those great discoveries which are made from time to time for the depopulation of the earth.") This treatment would cure not only yellow fever but also the political malady which afflicted the country. The result, Rush believed, would be an orderly national community governed by property owners for the benefit of "people of all classes, colors, and creeds."

Michal McMahon focuses on the aftermath of the epidemic and presents an "alternative version to the story of courageous physicians" battling the scourge of 1793. The most important response to the outbreak, McMahon argues, "was instead the struggles by city leaders and workers to ameliorate what they believed lay behind the periodic epidemics: a filthy urban environment and a dangerously polluted water supply." McMahon thus examines another aspect of community—the way in which Philadelphians unified after the epidemic to clean the city and to improve the urban environment. "Impelled by the devastation of the 1790s epidemics," Philadelphians continued to clean and pave the streets and, in the early nineteenth century, they invested in a costly and technologically sophisticated waterworks designed to pump the "pure" waters of the Schuylkill River to the city's inhabitants.

Philadelphia was known throughout the second half of the eighteenth century for its civic improvements, due in part to the legacy of the Quaker sense of communal responsibility. As the home of Benjamin Franklin, the city also reaped the harvest of his tremendous energy and intellect. Many inhabitants embraced both his scientific approach to knowledge and his deep commitment to enriching the community. Well before the Revolution, Philadelphians had established the Library Company of Philadelphia, the American Philosophical Society, and the University of Pennsylvania to advance philosophical, medical, and practical knowledge, and they supported a host of private and public measures designed to aid the needy, cure the sick, educate the children, clean and light the streets, combat the fires, and regulate the markets.[19]

Pragmatic reasons also animated Philadelphians to improve their physical setting. "Throughout the century," McMahon notes, the city "attended to urban environmental issues in response to epidemics." After the outbreak of yellow fever in 1741, for example, the colonial Assembly mandated that doctors visit arriving ships and confine sick passengers—who were believed to have introduced the fever—in a newly constructed lazaretto on an island in the Delaware River. The 1762 epidemic, according to McMahon, spurred the city "to organize the paving and cleaning of streets, removal of solid wastes, and extension of the city's drainage system." During the 1780s, the city government allocated money to enhance the center city blocks, paving more streets, hiring scavengers to clean the primary thoroughfares, and covering portions of Dock Creek.

Regardless of these efforts, in 1793 pigs, dogs, and rats roamed freely to feed on the garbage in the streets, especially in impoverished neighborhoods, while residents commonly disposed of their refuse and excrement in the alleys and gutters in front of their homes. The openings in sewers "exhale the most noxious effluvia," according to one contemporary, "for dead animals and every kind of nausea are thrown into them, and there remain till they become putrified."[20] Dock Creek continued to be a stagnant sludge of refuse in the center of the city. Not surprisingly, mortality during yellow fever outbreaks was extremely high among people who lived near the creek where mosquitoes thrived.

While Philadelphians debated the precise cause of the epidemics of the 1790s, many people embraced an environmental explanation for the disease. The epidemics thus were at least beneficial in forcing Philadelphians to act as a community in redoubling their efforts to clean the filthy urban environment. In addition to improving local conditions, Martin S. Pernick notes, Philadelphians also reformed their procedures for quarantining migrants arriving by ship.

Pernick's classic study of the epidemic traces how the controversies about the "causes of the disease, its proper treatment, and the conduct of those caught in the crisis" became entwined with diverse political and pragmatic issues. In arguments about the origins of yellow fever, city officials and the medical community generally "split along partisan political lines." Federalists, who loathed recent French refugees from Haiti for their support of the Democratic-Republicans, typically embraced the theory that immigrants introduced the disease to Philadelphia. Republicans, who supported French migration, usually detected a domestic source for fever; it sprouted in the unsanitary urban habitat. Business concerns also played a role in the response to the epidemic, as the city's merchants and other local boosters favored the "importation" theory.

Both newly-forming political parties exploited the epidemic for their own advantage and feared that their opponents would act likewise. Federalists believed that Republicans would manipulate the "domestic origins" argument to drive the United States Congress out of Philadelphia and to undermine cities in general. Indeed, after the epidemic, Thomas Jefferson concluded that "yellow fever will discourage the growth of great cities in the nation." Republicans suspected that the Federalist importation theory would hold special appeal for Americans imbued with deep patriotic feelings for the new nation. And they were right. The Federalists gained the most from the epidemic as they used it to widen the base of their new party.

Of course, political and pragmatic issues have, in both the past and present, influenced public policies and medical opinions. Debates about the origins of yellow fever and other scourges raged in Philadelphia long before 1793, and politics and economic interests frequently shaped proposals to control disease. In 1700, in response to the yellow fever epidemic of the previous year, Pennsylvania became the first colony to pass a law requiring all arriving ships with immigrants to be inspected. The yellow fever epidemic of 1741, as McMahon discusses, stimulated the governor and Assembly to support the construction of a "pest house" to quarantine sick immigrants on Province Island in the Delaware River. In 1754, after the death of more than 250 new arrivals, a team of doctors criticized the Assembly for not having passed "necessary regulations to prevent malignant Disease being generated by these People, after they came into Port."[21] The Assembly reacted, against the commercial interests of many merchants who trafficked in indentured servants and had close ties to the governor, by imposing stringent restrictions on vessels since "infectious Distempers have, notwithstanding previous laws, been introduced and spread in this province."[22] In addition, Benjamin Franklin and others often made overly optimistic claims about the health of colonial cities with pragmatic economic considerations in mind, for unhealthy conditions discouraged business and trade. Franklin may well have stopped publishing

Philadelphia's burial statistics in his newspaper because of his advertisers' concern for possible adverse effects on the city's economy.[23]

Pernick also calls our attention to the bitterness which many who stayed in the city felt toward those who fled. Republicans numbered disproportionately among relief workers during the epidemic, and they offered harsh criticism of citizens, especially wealthy ones, who abandoned their responsibilities during the time of crisis. For some Philadelphians, the decision to stay or flee was a moral one. Benjamin Garrigues, a Quaker carpenter who survived the 1798 epidemic, pondered this issue in his diary: "May this, O my Soul, lead thee to examine on what ground thou stands, and however it may be the lot of any to either stay here and suffer with the sufferers, or remove with those who may be indulged with that liberty, remember that no man is thy pattern." Garrigues decided to remain in the city to aid his friends and neighbors.[24]

Studying the 1793 epidemic permits scholars to gain insights into the history of the new nation, especially its urban centers. But people like Benjamin Garrigues challenge us on a different level to probe the morality of our own behavior in regard to the present global epidemiological threat. As individuals and as a society, whose example will we follow? Will we abandon our responsibility like those who bolted Philadelphia during the epidemic? They not only turned their back on their community to preserve their own lives, but, since most refugees feared that yellow fever was contagious, they also endangered the lives of people living in towns and villages to which they flew. Will we behave like those Philadelphians who shut themselves in their homes and refused to respond to the cries for help from their neighbors? Or will we act like the ordinary and extraordinary men and women who came to the aid of their relatives, friends, and community?

Finally, we also study the 1793 epidemic as a way to honor the officials, common citizens, and doctors (most of whom stayed in the city) who struggled courageously against the disease. Their doomed but heroic efforts to discover the cause of and a successful treatment for yellow fever constitute a true human tragedy. Their crusade represents the best of what it is to be human.

Let me conclude by quoting from Albert Camus' great novel, *The Plague*, an eloquent celebration of humankind's contest with evil, as represented by disease. Camus' fictional doctor wrote the story of the pestilence in order

> to bear witness in favor of those plague-stricken people, so that some memorial of the injustice and outrage done them might endure; and to state quite simply what we learn in a time of pestilence: that there are more things to admire in men than to despise. None the less, [the doctor] knew that the tale he had to tell could not be one of a final victory. It

could be only the record of what had had to be done, and what assuredly would have to be done again in the never ending fight against terror and its relentless onslaughts . . . by all who, while unable to be saints, still refuse to bow down tô pestilence and strive their utmost to be healers.[25]

In our own trying times, filled with horrors from yellow fever to AIDS, this is among the most important lessons to be learned from Philadelphia's epidemic, and one of the major reasons for commemorating that event.

NOTES

1. Edwin B. Bronner, ed., "Letter from a Yellow Fever Victim: Philadelphia, 1793," *Pennsylvania Magazine of History and Biography* 86 (1962): 205–207.
2. Laurie Garrett, *The Coming Plague: Newly Emerging Diseases in a World Out of Balance* (New York: Penguin Books, 1994).
3. Alfred W. Crosby, *Ecological Imperialism: The Biological Expansion of Europe, 900–1900* (Cambridge: Cambridge University Press, 1986), chapters 6 and 9.
4. The statistics are from Susan E. Klepp's essay in this volume. This and the following paragraphs draw both on that essay and on Klepp, "Zachariah Poulson's Bills of Mortality, 1788–1801," in Billy G. Smith, ed., *Life in Early Philadelphia: Documents from the Revolutionary and Early National Periods* (University Park: Pennsylvania State Press, 1995), pp. 221–223. See also Klepp, ed., *The Demographic History of the Philadelphia Region, 1600–1860* (Philadelphia: American Philosophical Society, 1989), pp. 103–111; and Billy G. Smith, *The "Lower Sort": Philadelphia's Laboring People, 1750–1800* (Ithaca: Cornell University Press, 1990), pp. 46–53.
5. Klepp, "Zachariah Poulson's Bills of Mortality," p. 221.
6. On medical knowledge and treatments, see the essay by J. Worth Estes in this volume.
7. Alexander Graydon, *Memoirs of His Own Time with Reminiscences of the Men and Events of the Revolution*, ed. John Stockton Littel (Philadelphia: Lindsay and Blakiston, 1846), p. 365; and Mathew Carey, *A Short Account of the Malignant Fever, Lately Prevalent in Philadelphia* (1794; reprint, New York: Arno Press, 1970), pp. 16–17, 21–22, 77.
8. Carey, *Short Account*, p. 27. The names and occupations of the decedents are given on pp. 121–163. Carey claimed that the "*filles de joie*" were particularly susceptible to epidemics because the "wretched debilitated state of their constitutions rendered them an easy prey to this dreadful disorder, which very soon terminated their miserable career" (ibid., p. 27). Elizabeth Drinker also observed that the fever predominated in the poorer sections of town; Elizabeth Evans, ed., *Weathering the Storm: Women of the American Revolution* (New York: Scribner, 1975), p. 179. See also Smith, "*Lower Sort*," pp. 52–56.
9. "A Useful Hint," *Mercury Daily Advertiser*, 19 August 1797.

10. Carey, *Short Account*, p. 27. Yellow fever deaths in streets, alleys, and lanes are recorded in Edmund Hogan, *The Prospect of Philadelphia and Check on the Next Directory* (Philadelphia: Printed by Francis and Robert Bailey, 1795).
11. Smith, *"Lower Sort,"* pp. 27–37.
12. Klepp, "Zachariah Poulson's Bills of Mortality," p. 222.
13. See Smith, *"Lower Sort,"* chapter 6.
14. Diary of Benjamin Garrigues, Historical Society of Pennsylvania, Philadelphia; *True American* (Philadelphia), 28, 30 September 1799, 8, 9 November 1799.
15. Bronner, ed., "Letter from a Yellow Fever Victim," p. 205.
16. Gary B. Nash, *Forging Freedom: The Formation of Philadelphia's Black Community, 1720–1840* (Cambridge, Mass.: Harvard University Press, 1988).
17. Ibid.
18. See Anthony F.C. Wallace, *The Death and Rebirth of the Seneca* (New York: Vintage, 1972).
19. See Smith, ed., *Life in Early Philadelphia*, chapter 1.
20. John K. Alexander, *Render Them Submissive: Responses to Poverty in Philadelphia, 1760–1800* (Amherst: University of Massachusetts Press, 1980), pp. 21–22. Quote from *Philadelphia Monthly Magazine*, August 1798, p. 69.
21. "A Colonial Health Report of Philadelphia, 1754," in *Pennsylvania Magazine of History and Biography*, 36 (1912): 479.
22. "Minutes of the Provincial Council," *Colonial Records of Pennsylvania*, 14 vols. (Harrisburg: T. Fenn & Co., 1851–1853), 6: 345.
23. Billy G. Smith, "Death and Life in a Colonial Immigrant City: A Demographic Analysis of Philadelphia," *Journal of Economic History* 37 (1977): 863, 874–75.
24. Diary of Benjamin Garrigues.
25. Albert Camus, *The Plague*, trans. Stuart Gilbert (New York: Random House, 1948), pp. 277–78.

Appendix I: "How Many Precious Souls Are Fled"?: The Magnitude of the 1793 Yellow Fever Epidemic

SUSAN E. KLEPP

T was a catastrophe; no one has doubted that. The Philadelphia yellow fever epidemic of 1793 killed thousands of inhabitants in three months. Just how great a catastrophe was a question that puzzled contemporaries and still puzzles historians. Statistical analysis of yellow fever mortality began early in the epidemic and was carried on throughout those deadly days in 1793. The lists compiled by dedicated ministers and health officials, and hurried into print by local publishers, have fascinated Philadelphians then and now. But those stark lists of the numbers of dead, sometimes classified by burial ground and by date of death, and more rarely by name, age, sex, occupation, cause of death, race, or residence, themselves bear mute testimony to a society in tatters. Lists are incomplete since some ministers, sextons, and officials fled the city or fell ill themselves. Other records were lost or misplaced. In the rush to bury the dead, burials went unrecorded or names, ages, and other details were forgotten. The published counts of deaths by burial ground and by cause often do not tally, for which both mathematical errors and typographical errors are responsible. Which are the right numbers? Some numbers can be checked against church registers or other records, but most cannot.

Judging the magnitude of the disaster requires two rather different assessments. One is to sort through the censuses, contemporary bills of mortality, reports of the Committee on the Malignant Fever (the precursor to the Board of Health), and other contemporary lists to try to arrive at approximately correct totals for the number of the dead and the proportion of the dead to the living. Philadelphia officials and publishers had been collecting annual data on deaths and births for over seventy years when the 1793 epidemic occurred, but never before had they responded to an epidemic with such an array of statistical information.[1] Daily weather reports, daily burials by burial ground, details of cause of death, the name, age, sex, and race of the deceased, and a census of the city were collected by publishers, churches, and government officials during the late summer and the autumn of 1793.[2] Perhaps the precision of numbers seemed to herald the eventual triumph of order and rationality. Perhaps the impersonality of arithmetic muted some of the horror at the loss of family, friends, and acquaintances. Certainly it was hoped that in quantifying the disaster some pattern—meteorological, residential, temporal, racial, or even religious—would emerge to point to an effective treatment, just as numbers had helped prove the effectiveness of smallpox inoculation in Boston earlier in the century.[3] The surviving lists often present very different numbers. Fortunately, the recent work of economists, demographers and quantitative historians makes the task of assessing these numbers easier than it would have been even a decade ago.

The other appraisal requires that this particular epidemic be compared to previous and subsequent epidemics in order to evaluate the apparent singularity of this disaster. This assessment will be more speculative: it demands both precise numbers for other times and places, which are often not available, as well as some conjectures about historical memory.

The population of the city of Philadelphia and its urbanized suburbs in mid-1793 was 51,200. Of this number, 47,880 (94 percent) were white and 3,320 (6 percent) were black. This decade saw a rapid increase in population, among the very largest in a century of spectacular growth.[4] The total number of residents increased from 44,096 in the first federal census of 1790 to 67,811 ten years later. Fertility rates had been falling since the peak years of the 1760s, but were still quite high. There were 24,915 individual births recorded in the city during the 1790s, producing an average crude birth rate of 46 births per thousand population.[5] In addition, thousands of immigrants arrived in the region and many intended to live in the city. More than 23,000 landed at the port of Philadelphia during the decade, while another 17,500 landed at Wilmington and completed their journey by land. Ireland and Germany contributed the largest share of the European immigrants, although refugees from France and its revolution were also a significant presence in the city. Other refugees, French colonials and their personal slaves, fled revolution in Saint Domingue. It was these ships arriving from the Caribbean in the summer of 1793 that were probably responsible for carrying yellow fever from Africa to the Caribbean to the north. There were also at least 3,600 African-American migrants who left rural areas for Philadelphia's comparative freedom and opportunity in this decade, nearly tripling the size of the black community in ten years. While thousands of Philadelphians died in 1793, they were replaced quickly. Over 6,000 immigrants had arrived in the region in 1792, and again in 1793. Yellow fever diverted some from a Philadelphia destination, but it did not diminish most immigrants' resolve, since over 4,000 arrived in the region in 1794 and unknown numbers of unrecorded migrants from neighboring ar-

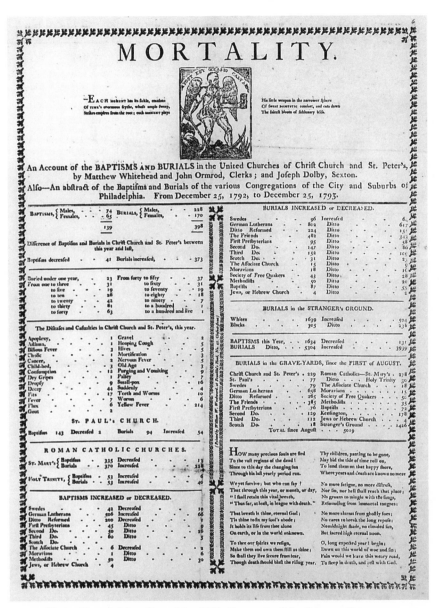

Christ Church Mortality table, 1793. Courtesy of the Library Company of Philadelphia.

eas sought business opportunities and housing in the temporarily depopulated city. Twenty-three hundred babies were born in 1793 and again in 1794, only slightly fewer than in previous years. By mid-1794 the population, despite yellow fever, is estimated at 53,600.[6]

Contemporary counts of annual mortality range from Zachariah Poulson's count of 4,992 (for 1 August 1793 to 1 August 1794) to the Christ Church bill of mortality list that adds up to 5,105, although the printed tally was 5,304 (for 25 December 1792 to 25 December 1793). These figures yield annual crude death rates between 93 and 104 per thousand population (or between 9 and 10 percent).[7] The most complete analysis of these error-ridden numbers is by Tom W. Smith. His estimate is 6,085 deaths for the calendar year, which produces an annual crude death rate of 119 (12 percent).[8] Estimates of annual white mortality range between 97 and 120 per thousand (10–12 percent). Estimates of annual black mortality range from 43 (certainly an undercount in Poulson's almanac) to between 92 and 102 per thousand population (9–10 percent).

Contemporary counts of deaths from yellow fever (actually all deaths from early August to November or December) range from the 3,293 deaths counted by the Committee on Malignant Fever to the perhaps imaginary figure of 5,019 presented in the Christ Church bill of mortality. The actual sum of the burials listed in the Christ Church bill for August through November comes to 4,134, not 5,019. Yet Tom W. Smith favors the higher number, as have others, based on an assumption that record-keeping broke down during the epidemic, even though precise figures cannot be found to support that 5,019 figure. Crude death rates during the epidemic would then fall between 64 and 98 per thousand population (6–10 percent).

These crude death rates during the epidemic are based on Philadelphia's total population. But many inhabitants fled during the epidemic and were therefore no longer at risk, since the infected mosquitoes did not fly far from the dock area. The resident population was estimated to have fallen to 24,675 persons in mid to late November 1793, based on a census of the city and suburbs. The census takers counted 3,293 deaths, making the crude yellow fever death rates of the at-risk population climb to 131 (13 percent). But asking residents to report the number of deaths will always produce an undercount since individuals who left no survivors or whose families subsequently fled will not be included. If there were in fact 5,019 yellow fever deaths, then the crude death rate rises to 203 (20 percent, or one death in every five persons presumably exposed to the disease). Since over forty percent of the white population was under 16 years of age and less likely to have fatal cases, the risk to resident adults could have been substantially higher. These may be high range estimates, since not all who fled left immediately and therefore the at-risk population was larger at the beginning of the epidemic, although many who fled had certainly returned by the time the census was finished—several weeks after the number of daily deaths began to diminish.

How accurate was the diagnosis of yellow fever? It has already been noted that all deaths from August to December were lumped together as yellow fever. But nearly one in four deaths recorded at Gloria Dei Swedish Lutheran Church from 20 July through December was attributed to causes other than yellow or malignant fever. Consumption and decay took their toll. A thirty-four-year-old woman died in childbirth, a thirty-year-old man fell from a haystack. Children succumbed to endemic diseases like infantile cholera, whooping cough, and smallpox. Worms and premature birth also afflicted the very young. Three of the yellow fever victims were noted to have been quite ill before the epidemic, so that yellow fever may only have been the proximate cause of death. Still, the 18 deaths attributed to other causes, plus the three very ill victims, are well above the number of deaths in the parish for the same months in previous years. In particular, "decay" and infant deaths were reported more frequently during the epidemic. Among the Episcopalians, annual lists of cause of death in 1793 and in subsequent epidemic years included an unusually high number of deaths from "fits" (often the product of high fever in infants and children), and teething and worms (deaths coinciding with weaning which might be from any cause). Either yellow fever was particularly likely to be under-reported among infants or there was a breakdown in childcare because of a combination of parental debility, women's other nursing responsibilities, a rise in unsanitary conditions, temporary unemployment, or food shortages. Similar factors may have affected the chronically ill, as well. The epidemic undoubtedly had both direct and indirect effects on the health and longevity of residents.

African Americans were probably more exposed to the infected mosquitoes than any other group in the city, since they assumed, both voluntarily and for wages, the responsibilities no one else would—they were the nurses, carters of the sick and dead, gravediggers, housecleaners, and guardians of the warehouses, stores, and residences abandoned by wealthier, white Philadelphians. The 1793 census reveals that one in four white Philadelphians had fled the city by November, but fewer than one in ten black residents departed.

African Americans did experience lower death rates in comparison to European Americans, perhaps because of some innate resistance, but certainly because a sizable minority had been born in the South, in Africa, or in the Caribbean where yellow fever was more common. Of African Americans married at Gloria Dei Church, 34 percent had fairly recently come from the southern states or from the Caribbean or Africa; of black mariners in 1803, 28 percent were born in those areas.[9] These immigrants were therefore more likely to have immunity from previous exposure. Contemporaries like Dr. Benjamin Rush were not entirely wrong in their early assumption of black imperviousness to yellow fever, although they obviously erred in jumping to a racial characterization of yellow fever risk rather than adopting a place-of-origin argument which would have included some immune Caribbean whites as well.[10] In fact, the notion that some individuals were "seasoned" to specific diseases by reason of their residence in countries where those diseases were prevalent was widely accepted at the time, which makes the race argument of 1793 all the more curious.

There were 22,929 resident whites counted in the November census of the city and suburbs, but only 1,746 blacks. The latter figure is certainly an undercount since black live-in servants were not separately enumerated—adding 400 persons raises the number to 2,142 resident African Americans, which corresponds to white reporting rates of 79 percent.[11] With yellow fever deaths apportioned at 3,095 for whites and 198 for blacks, by assuming that the annual proportions of deaths by race apply as well to the months of the epidemic, then the crude yellow fever death rates by race are 135 for at-risk whites and 92 for at-risk blacks (14 and 9 percent). This very rough calculation brings the Philadelphia experience with yellow fever mortality somewhat closer to the experiences of southern cities in the nineteenth century where large differences by race were the norm.[12] It is nonetheless the case that the true proportion of African American deaths will remain unknown because the under-recording of black deaths occurs in all the surviving documents from 1793, and because there is no separate listing of black deaths during the epidemic months. The uses of annual proportions of deaths by race are not necessarily trustworthy guides to racial differences during the epidemic since the cold weather diseases of the pulmonary system—pleurisy, tuberculosis, influenza—were most fatal to African Americans, followed by smallpox and measles, while white rates normally peaked during the heat of the summer as diarrheal and insect-borne diseases took their toll.[13] Higher black death rates may have occurred in the winter or spring, not during the epidemic. There had been an unusually high number of smallpox deaths reported just prior to the appearance of yellow fever.

In the early years of the nineteenth century, when some cases of yellow fever occurred in every year and epidemics were reported in 1802 and 1805, the seasonal patterns of adult black and white deaths were strikingly different. Black adult deaths were actually at their annual low during the peak epidemic months of August, September, and October, an indication that many Philadelphia African Americans had acquired innate immunity to yellow fever. White adult mortality peaked during the height of the yellow fever epidemics. Children of both races suffered from diarrhea during the hottest summer months. It was July and August that were most fatal to the youngest Philadelphians, not September and October when yellow fever dominated the mortality lists. If the same seasonal pattern by race prevailed in 1793, then the more precise estimate of the crude yellow fever death rate of the at-risk

African American population would be 32 per thousand, one-fourth the white rate. If figures were available for French colonials in the city, the result would undoubtedly be a similarly low rate. Mathew Carey noted in passing that "the French settled in Philadelphia, have been in a very remarkable degree exempt," but he did not link this observation to any larger theory of ethnic difference as he, and others, had done with African Americans.[14] The primary reason for differential mortality was that some people had immunity by virtue of previous exposure or innate resistance.

Age and sex factors were also present. Infants and children tend to have mild cases of yellow fever. In non-epidemic years, 39 percent of Episcopalian deaths were adults between 20 and 60 years old, but in the epidemic years of the 1790s that figure rose to 55 percent. The Episcopalians were relatively wealthy, and many had the wherewithal to flee to the countryside. At Gloria Dei Lutheran Church, serving a substantially poorer population of young transients and immigrants, the proportion of adult deaths rose from 23 percent to 56 percent between 1792 and 1793. Orphans, invalids, and the elderly were left without family support as these epidemics seemed perversely to single out the most productive residents, but not their dependents. It was particularly the nominal breadwinners who suffered high mortality. White males in 1793 had a crude annual death rate of 116 (based on all residents August to August 1793/4), white females 78, compared to 30 and 27 the year before.[15] While the death rate of white females nearly tripled in 1793, the rate for white males almost quadrupled.

Seasonal Deaths by Race and Age, Philadelphia, 1802–1805

| | *Percent distributions* | | | |
| | *Black* | | *White* | |
	Adults	*Children*	*Adults*	*Children*
August–October	17.3	28.2	36.5	39.6
November–January	28.7	14.1	22.8	16.3
February–March	21.8	23.9	22.2	13.8
May–July	32.2	33.8	18.5	30.3
Total	100.0	100.0	100.0	100.0
Base Number	87	71	2,353	2,466

Source: Philadelphia Board of Health, in Klepp, "The Swift Progress of Population": A Documentary and Bibliographic Study of Philadelphia's Growth, 1642–1859 (Philadelphia: American Philosophical Society, 1991), pp. 54–57. Churched populations only, seasons standardized to contain an equal number of days.

I have not found any convincing arguments for these sex differentials which characterize all outbreaks of yellow fever, in Philadelphia or elsewhere. It may be that more women than men left town during the epidemic. This had long been a practice among the wealthiest Philadelphians—women spent the summers at their country estates while their husbands continued to work in the fevers and agues of the city. But whether the average Philadelphia woman followed a similar plan in 1793 is unknown. Certainly the census of November 1793 found abandoned houses rather than solitary husbands in residence. And contemporaries described the desperate flight of whole families, burdened with as many of their belongings as possible, on the roads out of town. It is possible that men's outdoor occupations exposed them more often to infected mosquitoes, but in an era before screened windows, staying indoors would not have provided any protection against the rainbarrel and flowerpot-loving *Aedes aegypti* mosquitoes. In any event, all but the wealthiest women spent time outdoors marketing, fetching water, chopping kindling, hanging laundry, and, at least until the height of the epidemic, sociably sitting in the evenings at their front doors.

Contemporaries blamed dissipation for the sex differences, implying that men's greater tendency to drunkenness, overeating, and a "loose and abandoned way of living" predisposed them to illness.[16] This supposition cannot be tested. Immigrant status was a known factor in differential mortality during the southern epidemics of yellow fever in the nineteenth century, and since more men than women were recent migrants from Europe, then sex differences actually were the consequence of differential immigrant status. But since yellow fever had been absent from Philadelphia for 31 years, and because the 1762 outbreak was supposed to have been limited in space and time, few native Philadelphians would have acquired immunity from previous exposure. The scarce data on the age of the deceased in 1793 does not indicate any benefit to those over age 31. Both immigrant males from Europe and native-born females were unlikely to have the benefit of previous exposure to yellow fever.[17] The cause of sex differentials is unknown.

The poor were certainly at much greater risk of death, but it was not because of any moral failing, as J. H. C. Helmuth of the German Lutheran Church was at pains to point out to his readers. Rather, it was because they could not afford to flee and were more exposed to risk.[18] Carey estimated that seven-eighths of the dead were poor, an assertion which is supported by other evidence, although Carey's claim that this was due to "their neglect of cleanliness and decency" is unfounded.[19] Viruses acquired by the bite of mosquitoes are not destroyed by soap and water, still less by refined manners. Contemporary accounts would indicate that poverty had some effect on case rates, through debility caused by poor diets and over-work, and the inability of the poor to afford adequate nursing. Without constant nursing care, feverish patients could suffer from dehydration, malnutrition, and unsanitary conditions which would reduce the chances of recovery. Contemporary accounts detail the scarcity of nurses as well as the cries for water of solitary patients. The lists, censuses, and counts of the dead, as imperfect as they were, did clearly identify poverty as a factor in yellow fever deaths and pointed to two reasonably effective prophylactic measures—nursing care and flight. The hospital became less of a death trap once regular nursing was provided. The wealthy who fled Philadelphia survived, the poor who stayed died. In subsequent epidemics, hospitals were established early in the epidemics and tent cities were provided at a distance from the port which gave the poor a place to go. These measures probably prevented a repetition of the full horror of 1793.

The yellow fever epidemics were spectacular, but were just one disease factor in a society that would be considered, by late twentieth-century standards, in the midst of several epidemiological crises. In 1788 and in 1792–1799, yellow fever caused 18 percent of deaths among Episcopalians, but other acute infectious diseases (smallpox, whooping cough, and fevers) caused 21 percent of deaths, and "consumption" and "decay" (mostly tuberculosis) 28 percent of deaths. Convulsions, diarrhea, and other common causes of infant death accounted for another 21 percent of the total. Degenerative, accidental, maternal and other deaths accounted for the balance of Episcopalian deaths. The members of Christ Church and St. Peter's Episcopal parishes tended to be relatively wealthy, well-established Philadelphians. Gloria Dei Swedish Lutheran Church served the poorest population in Philadelphia. Southwark was a working class district with a high percentage of immigrants, sailors, dock workers, and young, struggling families. Infant deaths were more prominent there than in the Episcopalian churches both because there were more young couples bearing children and because unsanitary conditions, over-crowding, and poor diets disadvantaged the most vulnerable. Yellow fever raged in this suburb both because of poverty and because of proximity to the docks.

The epidemic of 1793 ravaged Philadelphia, afflicting young and middle-aged adults, the poor, men, and native-born or European-born whites, in particular. Yet the epidemic of 1793 was not the worst single epidemic in Philadelphia's history—either proportionately or absolutely. In 1699, an outbreak of yellow fever raised the annual death rate to 153 per thousand of the total white population (15 percent). Philadelphia was then a rustic village on the periphery of the English empire, it had no newspaper, and the proprietary government hushed up the health crisis. The future development of the fledgling colony depended on immigrants and investors, who would have been discouraged by news of a demographic disaster. Then in two months in 1918, 13,000 Philadelphians died during the pandemic of influenza. That epidemic seems to have been dwarfed by the carnage of World War I, as well as by the fact that the victims were disproportionately the young, the old, the ill, or soldiers and others in the camps. Neither epidemic is remembered, even

Assigned Causes of Death, 1790s

	Christ Church		Gloria Dei	
	Number	*Percent*	*Number*	*Percent*
Infancy and Childhood	377	21.1	230	39.9
Accident and Trauma	22	1.2	28	4.8
Yellow Fever	322	18.0	143	24.8
Other Infectious Disease (acute)	376	21.0	39	6.8
Other Disease (lingering)	498	27.9	93	16.1
Old Age	103	5.8	4	0.7
Miscellaneous	89	5.0	40	6.9
Total	1,787	100.0	577	100.0

Notes: In the eighteenth century, very few separate disease entities were recognized. Symptoms rather than specific diseases tended to be listed as the causes of death. Officials of the two churches used somewhat different categories, but the major diseases in each category in descending order of importance are: Infancy and Childhood: purging and vomiting, fits, teething and worms, flux, hives (croup); Infectious Disease (acute): fever, smallpox, bilious fever, nervous fever, bilious colic, pleurisy; Other Disease (lingering): decay, dropsy, consumption; Old Age: old age, palsy, apoplexy; Miscellaneous: childbed, mortification, inflammation, gravel.

by professional historians. The most recent history of Philadelphia devoted 11 of its 751 pages to the epidemic of 1793, two pages to the 1798 reoccurrence, and then referred back to these disasters on five other occasions. Neither the 1699 yellow fever epidemic nor the 1918 influenza epidemic merited inclusion.[20] Historical memory can be highly selective.

The decade of the 1790s was not the worst in the city's history despite the reappearance of yellow fever in 1797, 1798, and 1799. From 1690 to 1759, deaths exceeded births, and decadal death rates, bolstered by scores of epidemics of smallpox, measles, typhus, typhoid fever, scarlet fever, whooping cough, diphtheria, influenza, yellow fever, and other diseases, surpassed the rates of the last decade of the century. In the 1790s, the mean crude death rate was somewhere between 40 and 45 per thousand population, depending on which estimates are used. But crude death rates had averaged 46 per thousand for the entire 70-year period lasting from 1690 to 1759. Three of those decades experienced average death rates above 50 per 1,000—the 1690s, 1740s, and 1750s. Nor was Philadelphia's experience with yellow fever the worst in the nation's history. The Southern outbreaks of 1853 and 1878 were proportionately as bad or worse, with death rates running between 9 to 13 percent of the urban populations. In terms of absolute numbers of victims, the Southern epidemics were far worse, killing up to 20,000 individuals.[21]

It was recent improvements in health and longevity that helped to highlight the Philadelphia epidemic of 1793, not solely its absolute magnitude. Demographic shifts, including a growing proportion of native-born residents and falling birthrates, contributed to an appearance of improved health by reducing the proportion of those residents—immigrants and infants—with the highest probabilities of morbidity and mortality. Cultural changes that produced better childcare and led to more vegetables and less alcohol in the diet might have contributed to longevity. In addition, the end of the century saw more concern over personal cleanliness, greater attention to public sanitation, and an expanding water supply which allowed the cleansing of streets as well as of clothing and bodies. Local and state governments had implemented stronger quarantine procedures, and private and public organizations provided improved access to medical services. Subsidized medical care for poorer residents, especially free smallpox inoculation and midwifery services, had eliminated major smallpox epidemics and was reducing maternal mortality rates.[22]

Contemporaries calculated a Philadelphian's life expectancy at birth at just 13 years during the entire 36-year period from 1754 to 1790, which rose to an estimated 19 years during the eight years following the Revolution, 1782–1790. Life expectancy for the total population rose again to 26 years by 1814 (despite yellow fever) and for Episcopalians, who were wealthier than the average resident, to 31 years. During the first half of the nineteenth century, 1806–1868, all Philadelphians could expect to live an average of 35 years, while Quakers, both wealthier and more temperate than most, could look forward to 44 years.[23] Death rates had been falling since the 1760s, and the decline was especially pronounced after the Revolutionary War. While crude death rates had averaged 50 per thousand in the years immediately prior to the Revolution, crude death rates were down to 29 per thousand in the 1780s and 25 per thousand in the five years prior to the yellow fever epidemic. So 1793 stood out in part because it provided a sharp contrast to recent developments in health and longevity.

Philadelphia was a metropolis by 1793. It was the capital of the still-new United States, and internationally important as a symbol of revolutionary republicanism. The improvements in public health had been noticed by Philadelphians and especially by some enthusiastic supporters of the American and French revolutions who tied good health and the revolutionary state together. William Barton proclaimed in 1791 that a study of vital statistics proved that the United States possessed "an inherent, radical and lasting source of national vigor and greatness," deriving in large measure from "the benign influence of our government," and "the virtuous and simple manners of the great body of our inhabitants."[24] If health and the success of the

Table of Annual Philadelphia Crude Death Rates, 1690–1994:

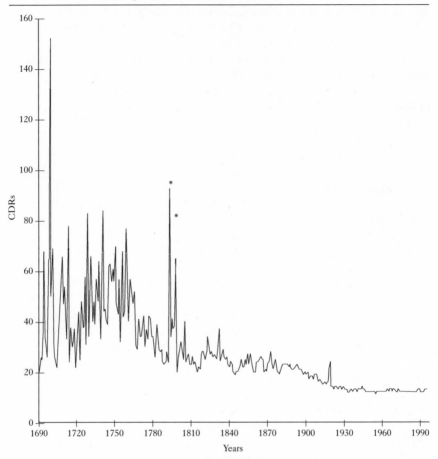

Deaths to 1807 based on local bills of mortality collected in Klepp, *"The Swift Progress of Population"*: *Documentary and Bibliographic Study of Philadelphia's Growth, 1642–1859* (Philadelphia: American Philosophical Society, 1991), and supplemented by church registers and other records. African American deaths are unavailable prior to 1720. From 1807 to the present, deaths have been recorded by the Department of Public Health, under slight changes of name and in various formats. My thanks to Warner Tillack of the Division of Vital Statistics for calculating the 1994 rate especially for this publication. The population base, prior to the reorganization of the health office in 1860, is the city of Philadelphia and its contiguous, urbanized suburbs. After 1860, the base is Philadelphia County. Before 1790, the calculations of P.M.G. Harris, "The Demographic Development of Colonial Philadelphia in some Comparative Perspective," *Proceedings of the American Philosophical Society* 133 (1989): 274, and Billy G. Smith, "Death and Life in a Colonial Immigrant City: A Demographic Analysis of Philadelphia," *Journal of Economic History* 37 (1977): 865, are used as the base population. Asterisks indicate the highest of the recent estimates for annual mortality in 1793 and 1798, while the solid line is based on contemporary reports. Special estimates are based, in part, on the work of Tom W. Smith.

Revolution were linked, then the sudden appearance of yellow fever in the nation's capital signalled a moral and political failure as well as a medical crisis. It was a symbolically important event in the nation's history. Various authors sought religious, political, or moral messages in the crisis of 1793. Both contemporaries and later commentators discovered larger meanings for the epidemic, sometimes through hyperbole. A centennial history of the United States pondered at length the appearance of "one of the most direful scourges that ever was known in the western world," so soon after "the founding of the republic" in a city known for "order, cleanliness, and temperance." The same author summarily dismissed in a few words the 1853 epidemic of yellow fever at New Orleans, "an oft-doomed city," even though more than twice as many died in New Orleans as in Philadelphia.[25] Perhaps it is telling that the most recent Philadelphia epidemic to capture the public's imagination, Legionnaires Disease, also afflicted patriotic Americans, this time during the celebration of the nation's bicentennial. It, too, seemed to signal an end to a period of optimism by countering "expectations that contemporary science is infallible and can solve all the problems that we can confront." Legionnaires Disease had no great impact on the city's or the nation's death rate, but it anticipated an era of AIDS, Ebola fever, Lyme disease, and other new and exotic plagues—some very serious, others less so.[26] The combination of national symbols and mysterious, perhaps foreign, diseases has continued to grab public attention and to focus wide-spread anxieties about both disease and national purpose.

What happened in Philadelphia as capital of the young republic was therefore eminently newsworthy and historically significant. In addition, Philadelphia had articulate men of science who were accustomed to expressing their views in print, learned societies that both stimulated research and preserved public and private papers relating to the epidemic, as well as novelists, journalists, and a competitive press anxious to expand sales. The simultaneous outbreaks of yellow fever in the smaller and more provincial cities of New York and Portsmouth received less attention. The equally devastating 1793 yellow fever epidemic at Harrisburg has long been forgotten, even though residents were far more aggressive in seeking out causes for the disaster and enacting public health measures than Philadelphians.[27]

Memory of the Philadelphia epidemic might have faded over time, as it did for Harrisburg's, but for another circumstance. J. H. Powell's 1949 book, *Bring Out Your Dead*, revitalized the prominence of Philadelphia's 1793 yellow fever epidemic.[28] Powell presented a dramatic, even melodramatic, story that has had considerable appeal to both specialists and non-specialists. There were two villains in his telling of the tale. One was the fever. The other was Dr. Benjamin Rush, whose supposedly irrational therapeutics represented a triumph of theory over reality. Rush was portrayed as surrounding himself with the adoring, frightened masses, while those who questioned his theory became enemy conspirators. On the other side were Powell's heroes. These were the pragmatic, middle-class managers who took over the administration of the city. Two world views were at war in Philadelphia in 1793, according to Powell. One side was dogmatic, demagogic, and destructive. The other was moderate, middle class, entrepreneurial, and constructive. Yellow fever had become a metaphor for the Cold War. Powell's epidemic was an allegory of ideological conflict with, however, a happy ending attached. The drama of his reconstruction of the event has shaped our understanding of public health in the city ever since, despite more dispassionate and sophisticated studies of the disease and the city.[29]

The 1793 epidemic was both terrifying and a terrible loss of human life. Up to 12 percent of the population died that year, and perhaps one in five of those exposed to the infected mosquitoes sickened and died. It was, however, just one of many deadly epidemics that struck the continental United States from the seventeenth through the early twentieth centuries. But more than most, this particular epidemic stands out in the collective memories of Americans. It struck able-bodied heads of families and left mourning widows, orphans, and aged parents in its wake. It appeared, given the lack of knowledge of immune reactions and a misreading even of the available evidence, to highlight racial divisions in America just as issues of slavery and freedom were being renegotiated. It devastated the nation's capital just five years after a new, experimental republican government had been established. The search for its meaning absorbed some of America's most prominent men—doctors, lawyers, government officials, writers, and publishers—and produced a vast literature and an array of statistics that continue to intrigue the general public and scholars in a number of disciplines. The attempt to capture the essential meaning, if any, of this one yellow fever epidemic persists. The search for ever more precise numbers also continued. By the early nineteenth century, the functions of 1793's almanac writers, newspaper publishers, church sextons, and hospital administrators were consolidated into the first Board of Health. Ever more elaborate lists of numbers framed public health policy, defined medical practice and uncovered moderately effective preventative measures—nursing, flight, and nuisance control. Neither numbers nor symbols captured those damned mosquitoes, however. That was a different story.

POSTSCRIPT

The following previously unpublished sheet provides an example of the fascination with numbers expressed by private citizens as well as by institutions, professionals, and publishers during the epidemic years of the late eighteenth and early nineteenth centuries.[30] Other examples might be found preserved in the collections of the American Philosophical Society, the College of Physicians of Philadelphia, the Library Company of Philadelphia, the Historical Society of Pennsylvania, and the Archives of the Pennsylvania Hospital. In this exercise, Quaker Cadwallader Evans has tried to find a pattern by linking mean daytime temperatures with subsequent epidemics, measured by the absolute numbers of deaths.[31] His methodology and assumptions may seem antiquated—there is no sophisticated statistical analysis here. His research did not establish a diagnostic tool for nineteenth-century public health officials. But despite the shortcomings of his assumptions and of his results, he may, inadvertently, have been on to something. The *Aedes aegypti* mosquito will not bite at temperatures below 67°. Cooler temperatures at three in the afternoon could easily have dropped below 67° at night, preventing the mosquitoes from biting sleeping victims, delaying egg production, and short-circuiting the cycles between vectors and hosts needed to sustain an epidemic of yellow fever in a northern climate. But the numbers alone would not predict the years when citizens should take flight from the city. A knowledge of disease transmission and of the habits of mosquitoes would be necessary. Published by the generous permission of the American Philosophical Society.

On the Yellow Fever.
I have employed some leisure hours at different times in endeavouring to ascertain what was the mean degree of heat at 3 PM only, by the Thermometer, in the months of June and July, in seventeen years 1793 to 1809 with a view to find some rule of determining every year before the end of July whether the Yellow fever would prevail here in that year or not: as it seems to be admitted by the Physicians that a certain degree of heat is essential to its commencement and progress, whether it is imported or originates here. I have taken by account of the State of the Thermometer from the observations of David Rittenhouse and his family, of Dr. Duffield and of the Board of health as published—and I find.

	the mean heat of June at 3 PM	the mean heat of July at 3 PM	average heat of the two months at 3 PM	mean heat of August at 3 PM	Remarks Note— *Yellow fever years are set down with red ink [here bold]*
1793	**79.7°**	**84.3°**	**82°**	**82.7°**	**Great yellow fever in Philadelphia 4000 died in 3 months.**
1794	75.6	80.4	78	81.7	No alarm of Yellow fever in Philada
1795	75	82.2	78.6	80.3	Ditto.—fever in N York & Norfolk
1796	76.5	81.5	79	80.3	no alarm here.
1797	**79**	**84.2**	**81.6**	**79**	**Yellow fever here— 1250 died in 3 months**
1798	**77**	**82**	**79.5**	**86.5**	**Great yellow fever here. 3500 died in 3 months**
1799	**77**	**84**	**80.5**	**82**	**Yellow fever—1000 died in 3 months**
1800	75	78	76.5	78	No alarm here—fever in Baltimore
1801	76	80	78	77	no alarm here
1802	**75.7**	**78**	**76.3**	**78**	**a little yellow fever here—very slight**
1803	**76.9**	**81.8**	**79.3**	**79.4**	**Fever here, but not bad**
1804	71	78	74.5	75	no alarm here
1805	**75**	**83**	**79**	**81**	**Fever bad only in Southwark after 1 Sept r**
1806	78.1	78.7	78.4	72.1	no alarm here
1807	71.6	77.9	74.7	75.2	Ditto
1808	75.5	78.8	77.1	76.5	Ditto
1809	73.7	75.1	74.4		

From this List, which I believe is correctly taken off, if we examine the fourth column, which contains the mean heat of June and July taken together, it seems, that the mean heat of 79 degrees is the dividing Line.—When the average heat of those two months taken together at 3 P.M. is below 79. there has been no alarm of yellow fever spreading here in Philadelphia, during that whole Season.—When above 79 it has always spread before the Season was over.—When exactly at 79. in 1796 it did not spread.—in 1805 it did spread. The only exception to the Rule seems to be in 1802 when there was a slight degree of the yellow fever here. This deviation I cannot account for.

In the present summer of 1809, June has been very cool, and July the coolest for 17 years past. and both months together about two degrees cooler even than in 1802. So that judging of the future by the Past, we may almost rest assured that the yellow fever will not prevail here this year:

Cadwr Evans

No 60 North 8th Street
July 31st 1809—

NOTES

1. My thanks to Dr. Margaret Humphreys for her most helpful comments on this article. On the rise of statistical analysis in this period, see James H. Cassedy, *Demography in Early America: Beginnings of the Statistical Mind, 1600–1800* (Cambridge, Mass.: Harvard University Press, 1969), and his *American Medicine and Statistical Thinking, 1800–1860* (Cambridge, Mass.: Harvard University Press, 1984). Also, Patricia Cline Cohen, *A Calculating People: The Spread of Numeracy in Early America* (Chicago: University of Chicago Press, 1982).

2. Major sources for statistics on the epidemic are Mathew Carey, *A Short Account of the Malignant Fever, Lately Prevalent in Philadelphia* (Philadelphia: Mathew Carey, 1793), which includes deaths from 1 August through 9 November 1793, by day and by church. He also provided a list of the names of the dead, drawn from church registers. *Committee on the Malignant Fever, Minutes of the Proceedings of the Committee, 1793, on the Malignant Fever* (Philadelphia: Crissy and Markly, 1848), p. 243, which gives the results of the census of Philadelphia by district, November 1793, counting the resident inhabitants and the number who had fled, by race, with the number of the dead. J. Henry C. Helmuth, *A Short Account of the Yellow Fever in Philadelphia, for the Reflecting Christian*, trans. Charles Erdmann (Philadelphia: Jones, Hoff & Derrick, 1794), pp. 21–22, 46–50, gives the most sophisticated contemporary account of differential mortality by age, sex, and social status. His analysis is the only one to seriously consider the characteristics of the populations at risk. Christ Church (Philadelphia), *An Account of the Baptisms and Burials [etc.] From December 25, 1792, to December 25, 1793* [Philadelphia, 1794], gives the annual deaths by burial ground and race; Episcopalian deaths by age, by sex, and by cause; and deaths from the 1st of August by burial ground. Note that the printed

totals exceed the sum of the individual items, and that for some burial grounds the number of deaths since August is higher than annual deaths. Zachariah Poulson, *Town and Country Almanac for the Year of Our Lord, 1795* (Philadelphia: Poulson, 1794), gives deaths by church, by race and by sex, 1 August 1793 to 1 August 1794. Black deaths are certainly under-reported. The latter two sources can be found in Susan E. Klepp, *"The Swift Progress of Population": A Documentary and Bibliographic Study of Philadelphia's Growth, 1642–1859* (Philadelphia: American Philosophical Society, 1991), pp. 52, 79. For population of the city and its contiguous suburbs, see United States Census Bureau, Department of State, Censuses of Pennsylvania for 1790, 1800. See also Billy G. Smith, *The "Lower Sort": Philadelphia's Laboring People, 1750–1800* (Ithaca: Cornell University Press, 1990), esp. pp. 51–53, 204–208.

3. See Lemuel Shattuck, "On the Vital Statistics of Boston," *American Journal of the Medical Sciences*, n.s., 1 (1841): 369–401.

4. Susan E. Klepp, *Philadelphia in Transition: A Demographic Study of the City and Its Occupational Groups, 1720–1830* (New York: Garland, 1989), p. 336.

5. Susan E. Klepp, "Zachariah Poulson's Bills of Mortality, 1788–1801," in *Life in Early Philadelphia*, ed. Billy G. Smith (University Park: Pennsylvania State Press, 1995), pp. 219–242.

6. Hans-Jürgen Grabbe, "European Immigration to the United States in the Early National Period, 1783–1820," in *The Demographic History of the Philadelphia Region, 1600–1860*, ed. Susan Klepp (Philadelphia: American Philosophical Society, 1989), Table 1, p. 192; Graph 2, p. 200; Klepp, "Zachariah Poulson's Bills of Mortality."

7. Crude death rates are the deaths per thousand population. These death rates are considered crude because they do not take into account the underlying age, sex, and ethnic composition of society. The earliest United States censuses did not include details of age and sex for all inhabitants so that the detailed characteristics of the underlying population are often unknown for the 1790s.

8. Tom W. Smith, "The Dawn of the Urban-Industrial Age: The Social Structure of Philadelphia, 1790–1830" (Ph.D. diss., University of Chicago, 1980), pp. 90–91.

9. K. David Patterson, "Yellow Fever Epidemics and Mortality in the United States, 1693–1905," *Social Science and Medicine* 34 (1992): 861–863. Kenneth F. Kiple and Virginia H. Kiple, "Black Yellow Fever Immunities, Innate and Acquired, As Revealed in the American South," *Social Science History* 1 (1977): 419–436. Immigrants calculated from Gloria Dei marriage records, 1793–1805, and in Gary B. Nash, *Forging Freedom: The Formation of Philadelphia's Black Community, 1720–1830* (Cambridge, Mass.: Harvard University Press, 1988), Table 3, p. 136.

10. Carey, *Short Account*, pp. 77–78, gives the contemporary view. Absalom Jones and Richard Allen, *A Narrative of the Proceedings of the Black People, during the Late Awful Calamity in Philadelphia in the Year 1793* (1794; reprint, Philadelphia: Independence National Historical Park, 1993). *Letters of Benjamin Rush*, ed. L. H. Butterfield, 2 vols. (Princeton: Princeton University Press, 1951), 2: 654–5, 658, 663, 674, 684, 731–2.

11. The 1793 census purports to count the number of dead, and the number of those who fled and those who stayed by race, but encompasses only 79 percent of whites and 67 percent of blacks according to the more thorough federal censuses.

12. See Patterson, "Yellow Fever Epidemics," pp. 861–863; Kiple and Kiple, "Black Yellow Fever Immunities," pp. 419, 424ff.
13. Klepp, "Seasoning and Society: Racial Differences in Mortality in Eighteenth-Century Philadelphia," *William and Mary Quarterly*, 3rd. ser., 51 (1994): 473–506.
14. Carey, *Short Account*, p. 75.
15. The sex ratio of African Americans was not queried in the federal censuses, but rough estimates can be calculated by applying the sex ratio of the white population to the African American population. This yields a crude death rate of 100 for African American males and 72 for females, compared to 40 and 30 in the previous twelve months. Deaths in 1793 were then two and a half times the previous year—an increase slightly below that experienced by white females.
16. Helmuth, *Short Account*, pp. 21–22; Carey, *Short Account*, p. 74.
17. William J. Hinke, *Pennsylvania German Pioneers*, 2 vols. (1934; reprint, Baltimore: Genealogical Publishing, 1966) is one of the few sources for computing the sex ratio of European immigrants.
18. Helmuth, *Short Account*, p. 47. He argued that yellow fever was a judgment on the entire city for not repenting, rather than a sign of individual sinfulness.
19. Carey, *Short Account*, p. 74.
20. Russell F. Weigley, ed., *Philadelphia: A 300-Year History* (New York: W.W. Norton, 1982), pp. 181–188, 190–192, 197–198, 201, 226, 230, 254, 738–739.
21. Patterson, "Yellow Fever Epidemics," pp. 855–865; Margaret Humphreys, *Yellow Fever and the South* (New Brunswick: Rutgers University Press, 1992).
22. See Klepp, *Philadelphia in Transition*, pp. 225–306.
23. William Barton, "Observations on the Probabilities of the Duration of Human Life, and the Progress of Population, in the United States of America," *Transactions of the American Philosophical Society* 3 (1793): 56, life tables for Philadelphia, 1754–1790 and 1782–1790; *An Address from the President and Directors of the Pennsylvania Company for Insurances on Lives and Granting Annuities* (Philadelphia: Maxwell, 1814), reprinted in Harrison S. Morris, *A Sketch of the Pennsylvania Company for Insurances on Lives and Granting Annuities* (Philadelphia: Lippincott, 1890), pp. 117–121, life expectancy in Philadelphia, circa 1814; Pliny Earle Chase, "Philadelphia Life Tables," *Proceedings of the American Philosophical Society* 11 (1869): 17–22, life expectancy in Philadelphia, 1806–1868; Tom W. Smith calculates a life expectancy of 31 years in 1830, "Dawn of the Urban-Industrial Age," p. 102; while Louise Kantrow finds that the very wealthy had life expectancies in the low 40s in the eighteenth century, and the high 40s or low 50s in the nineteenth, "Life Expectancy of the Gentry in Eighteenth and Nineteenth-Century Philadelphia," in *The Demographic History of the Philadelphia Region, 1600–1860*, pp. 312–327.
24. Barton, "Observations on the Probabilities of the Duration of Human Life," p. 26.
25. R. M. Devens, *Our First Century: Being a Popular Descriptive Portraiture of the One Hundred Great and Memorable Events of Perpetual Interest in the History of Our Country* (Springfield, Mass.: Nichols, 1878), pp. 515, 516.
26. See Gordon Thomas and Max Morgan-Witts, *Anatomy of an Epidemic* (Garden City, N.Y.: Doubleday, 1982), quote by David J. Sensor, Director of the Centers for Disease Control, on p. vi.

27. Carey, *Brief History*, p. 87, gives the death rate in Harrisburg as one-fifteenth of the population, equivalent to a crude death rate of 67 per thousand, and alludes to a similar outbreak in rural Delaware. An antiquarian account of the Harrisburg epidemic and of the public health measures undertaken, despite the strenuous objections of some property owners, is in George H. Morgan, comp., *Annals, Comprising Memoirs, Incidents, and Statistics of Harrisburg from the Period of Its First Settlement* (Harrisburg: Brooks, 1858), pp. 91–104.

28. J. H. Powell, *Bring Out Your Dead: The Great Plague of Yellow Fever in Philadelphia in 1793* (Philadelphia: University of Pennsylvania Press, 1993); earlier editions published by various publishers appeared in 1949, 1965, and 1970.

29. For more balanced views of Rush's medical theories, see the work of J. Worth Estes on yellow fever diagnostics in this volume; James C. Riley, *The Eighteenth-Century Campaign to Avoid Disease* (New York: St. Martin's Press, 1987), pp. 140–150, on Benjamin Rush, yellow fever and environmentalism; other essays in the present volume address additional issues that Powell dramatized.

30. American Philosophical Society, Ms. Coll. George Vaux Collection No. 73. 1809 July 31 Cadwallader Evans—Statement on Yellow Fever, tables of data.

31. There were two men named Cadwallader Evans: one was a merchant who lived from 1749–1821, the other was a surveyor and state assemblyman who lived from 1762–1841. The latter was related to the Rittenhouse family and so may be the author of this analysis. See Elaine F. Crane et al., eds., *The Diary of Elizabeth Drinker*, 3 vols. (Boston: Northeastern University Press, 1991), 3: 2145.

Appendix II: Yellow Fever Since 1793: History and Historiography[1]

MARGARET HUMPHREYS

THE story of yellow fever has become something of a growth industry in historical circles in recent years. As a disease, it fascinates historians for its drama, mortality, and ability to incite medical debate.
Yellow fever was a disease in the United States that demanded a
response from the community. It was never hidden or seen as part of life, like
tuberculosis, hookworm, and malaria might be. Yellow fever always created a
crisis when it appeared, thus illuminating the particular patterns of community organization and medical thought at the times of its onslaught. It also
spurred reform, as the futility of contemporary measures and concepts gave
way to new ideas and techniques.

The works in this volume focus on the first major yellow fever epidemic
in the United States, that which occurred in Philadelphia in 1793. This essay
will attempt to answer questions that may remain in the reader's mind at the
completion of the volume. What happened to yellow fever in the United
States after 1793? How and when did ideas about its etiology and prevention
change? Given the multiple historiographic viewpoints of these essays, how
do they fit into the broader historiography of this stimulating disease? And,
finally, what, if anything, remains to be said or done about yellow fever? I will
close my analysis with suggestions and speculation about further research.

THE HISTORY OF YELLOW FEVER IN
THE UNITED STATES

The early history of yellow fever in the United States was one of scattered epidemics accompanied by a brief flurry of medical response without the generation of new public health policy. Yellow fever visited the American colonies
intermittently during the colonial period but was not a major presence.[2] The
first epidemic to arouse widespread attention and alarm, the 1793 Philadelphia
epidemic, is well known to medical historians.[3] Although it aroused extensive

discussion about contagion and quarantine at the time, it had little lasting influence on public health practice. The medical consensus reached during that epidemic did establish anticontagionism as the ruling medical dogma about yellow fever transmission, and this was preached to the hordes of southern medical students educated at the Philadelphia medical school in the following decades. Likewise, epidemics that visited the republic during the first three or four decades of the nineteenth century caused flickers of reform impulse without creating hearty flames. Each epidemic was attended by calls for quarantine and cleanliness, with the advocates for each sparring inconclusively as their respective public health measures usually failed equally well.[4] This began to change by mid-century. In the two decades prior to the Civil War, New Orleans and the South were visited repeatedly by yellow fever, creating the critical energy for medical researchers and public health workers to take on the disease in earnest. By the 1850s yellow fever had become almost exclusively a southern disease. For reasons that are not entirely clear from its biology, yellow fever moved progressively southward over the course of the nineteenth century and finally disappeared from the country in 1905. Thus research on the disease was largely the province of physicians in the South; the medical centers of New York, Philadelphia, and Boston were little concerned by it after mid-century. Although the massive anticontagionist work on yellow fever written by René La Roche in 1855 was a Philadelphia product, his literature review form of analysis was already being challenged by the direct observations of obscure physicians in the rural South.[5]

A new epidemiological theory emerged from this ferment. The doctrine of transportability sidestepped issues of contagionism and anticontagionism by simply asserting that somehow or the other yellow fever traveled from place to place. Physician after physician in rural Louisiana, Mississippi, and South Carolina documented the arrival in their small towns of yellow fever by boat or train. The first case appeared after some sort of contact with an infected place, and then the disease spread through the town. The dissemination was often erratic—not house-to-house but jumping from one neighborhood to the next. They agreed person-to-person contagion seemed wrong, and accepted the standard wisdom on that score. Although they overtly expressed discomfort at going against the opinions of their Philadelphia professors, these physicians felt the overall pattern of transport from fever centers like New Orleans to outlying towns was too clear to deny. The disease might well be indigenous to New Orleans since it occurred so frequently there; their little towns on the other hand rarely saw it, so it was hard to argue that the disease should arise spontaneously this summer and not last.[6] The doctrine of transportability was accompanied by a seed-soil analogy that was to become standard in public health thinking for decades to come. Something was transported, but it seemed to require proper local conditions to become established. Southern physicians wedded some features of contagionism and anticontagionism by stating that the seed of the epidemic was brought from the disease center, but that if the soil was hostile to it the disease could not take root. They universally believed that filth fostered the seed (whatever it was), and that cleanliness would protect a town. This theory then generated a two-pronged approach to yellow fever prevention: quarantine *and* sanitation. The discovery of distinct bacterial organisms as the etiologic agents for tuberculosis, syphilis, cholera, and other diseases during the last quarter of the nineteenth century gave precision to the notion of an as-yet undiscovered germ without changing the basic structure of this argument and its concomitant public health implications.[7]

Necessary to the acceptance of the notion of transportability was the concept that yellow fever was a distinct disease. Most southern physician-authors accepted this notion by the 1850s, based on their direct experience with the disease. The opposing view claimed that yellow fever was merely an exacerbated form of malaria or the other endemic fevers. Its severity was due to the confluence of environmental factors acting on the body in concordance with the usual fever common to that locale. If cold, harsh winters made pneumonia more deadly, summers that were hot, long, and dry could breed particularly severe fevers. By mid-century many Southern physicians doubted this, saying instead that the symptom complex of yellow fever was so distinctive, and never seen in part, that it must be a separate disease with its own cause. They made long lists of the distinguishing features of the disease; in 1873, New Orleans physician J. C. Faget even identified a pathognomonic sign—a slow pulse in the setting of a high fever. Accepting that yellow fever was a disease in itself was essential to further understanding its behavior and modeling public health practices against it.[8]

The 1850s marked the appearance of public health advocates in the South. More than just physicians appointed to emergency boards of health during epidemics, these men took on public health issues with dedication in their careers and publications. This was particularly true in New Orleans, where the foundation of what was to become Tulane's School of Tropical Public Health was laid by such men as Stanford E. Chaillé in the 1850s. These public health advocates argued loudly for sanitation and sometimes for quarantine. Support for the latter waxed and waned in the 1850s as it had in earlier decades. While little actual progress was made toward public health reform, the institutions of boards of health began to assume some solidity; in earlier years the usual pattern had been for boards to coalesce during an epidemic and then fade away after the threat had passed.[9]

During the Civil War, yellow fever was remarkably absent. Southerners had predicted that the disease would kill off the invading Yankees, but it did not oblige. In contrast, the Yankees claimed that it was the military police and rigid sanitary action of, for example, the occupying army of New Orleans, which kept yellow fever away. It appeared that the South could prevent yellow fever, if only the proper steps were taken.[10]

In the immediate postbellum period, the South suffered only scattered outbreaks of yellow fever, the worst being in 1872 and 1873. During the 1870s, in spite of that decade's depression, commercial activities revived from their Reconstruction doldrums. Railroad lines were laid or restored throughout the South, connecting its tropical ports to the hinterland. Shippers established new trading agreements with the Caribbean, Mexico, and South America for the importation of bananas, coffee, sugar, and other produce. New Orleans again became a central port, and the imported goods were unloaded into railroad cars to be taken deep into the country's interior.[11] The resumption of trade brought renewed opportunities for disease transmission from tropical ports while at the same time supplying the disease with easy transport inland. In 1878, disaster struck. A severe yellow fever epidemic in New Orleans quickly spread along rail and water lines to one hundred cities and towns in the Mississippi and Ohio River valleys. One estimate cited nearly a hundred thousand cases and twenty thousand deaths in the warm months of 1878. The economic toll was staggering as well, as commerce was frozen throughout the South. In 1879, yellow fever occurred again, with lesser severity.[12]

For the first time politicians, editors, and physicians turned to the federal government for help in controlling yellow fever. With Reconstruction just past, Congress was in the habit of believing the South could not take care of itself and required federal guidance and assistance. The Southern disease had reached into Ohio and Illinois with promise of worse behavior on its next return. The South appeared to be doing a very poor job of preventing the disease which now threatened the national health. Commercial interests in New York and Philadelphia urged Congress to take charge of the situation so the economic losses of 1878 would not be repeated.[13]

Congress created the National Board of Health in March of 1879. Its governmental location reflected its purpose: it was part of the Treasury Department and authorized under the constitutional power of the federal government to regulate interstate commerce. The founding members of the National Board were empowered mainly to organize quarantines and only indirectly to assist state and local boards with sanitation. The seed/soil doctrine still held sway; the members of the National Board of Health were strong sanitationists who, ironically, were to devote the major part of their undertaking to the establishment of a "scientific" quarantine.

In the writings and actions of the National Board of Health, quarantine assumed a new form. During the antebellum period, quarantine had been merely a period of detention determined arbitrarily to be anywhere from a few days to a month or more. Supposedly this wait would insure that all contagious persons on board would have declared themselves. A new technique was suggested by the transportability theory's seed/soil analogy. If the seed could be killed, and the soil rendered inhospitable, then yellow fever could be stopped. By the 1880s it was widely believed that the cause of yellow fever could be eradicated by disinfectants, leaving aside the question of whether the disinfectant was neutralizing a poisonous air or killing the responsible microorganism. The disinfectants chosen tended to be sulphurous acid gas for the holds of ships and the walls of railroad cars, heat for items of clothing, and chloride solutions for anything else that needed washing down. Accordingly, quarantine stations became disinfection points, with a delay of only a few days as the process was carried out. Sick passengers were detained in the station's hospitals, but those with no sign of disease after the detention period of a few days were allowed through.[14]

The National Board of Health carried out a variety of programs in the South, including organizing rail quarantines around Memphis and New Orleans during the 1879 epidemics, conducting sanitary surveys of southern cities, and establishing maritime quarantine stations for the Gulf Coast. However, when yellow fever failed to return in 1880, 1881, and 1882, Congress lost interest in the National Board and canceled its funding. The members of the board had hoped to establish a national beacon for public health reform but its fate was too closely tied to an unpredictable disease. Its job had been created out of economic need, not a congressional conviction favoring the ideals of the board's members. Lack of political savvy and infighting among public health leaders contributed to the board's demise as well.[15]

Yellow fever reappeared in a dramatic fashion next in 1888, followed by epidemics in 1892 and 1897–99. Again federal action was demanded, and again Congress responded. This time, though, it was an obscure entity known as the Marine Hospital Service which took charge. This federal agency ran small hospitals in the nation's ports whose function was to care for the sailors of the merchant marine. Since charity hospitals often limited their care to local inhabitants, these itinerant workers required a special locus for hospitalized care, provided by the federal system. During the decade of the 1880s, the director of the Marine Hospital Service saw the opportunity for expanding his powers, and seized it. He argued that since the Marine Hospital Service already had a base in each of the port cities, it was ideally suited to take on quarantine responsibilities as well. The Marine Hospital Service built or acquired quarantine stations along the Gulf and Atlantic coasts, charged with the task of excluding yellow fever. With each late nineteenth-century epidemic, the service acquired more funding and power. Finally, in 1902, the name was changed to the United States Public Health Service in recognition of the broadened scope of the agency's activities. Concern with cholera, smallpox, and immigration all played a role in generating the perception that such a service was needed, but it was yellow fever that mainly built the United States Public Health Service into an enduring entity of federal public health action.[16]

After the Spanish-American War led to U.S. domination of Cuba, the surgeon general sent a commission of army officers, headed by Walter Reed, to study yellow fever there. In 1900, Reed and his co-workers established the mosquito vector of yellow fever.[17] Once accepted, the theory provided a strikingly new basis for yellow fever prevention and control. William Crawford Gorgas' application of the theory to Panama, allowing American workers to finally complete the Canal, is the stuff of legend.[18] Less well known is its use in the last United States yellow fever epidemic, which occurred in 1905. The United States Public Health Service invaded New Orleans with scores of workers armed with anti-mosquito zeal. They sprayed houses with insecticide, oiled cisterns and other pools of fresh water to suffocate larvae, and screened houses. School children were rewarded for each mosquito killed and collected. Overall the service was able to report a mortality rate less than expected and an early end to the epidemic. Modern public health had triumphed.[19]

Although yellow fever never returned to the United States, its history was fundamentally influenced elsewhere by an American institution. The Rockefeller Foundation, after funding projects on hookworm and malaria in the southern United States during the second decade of the twentieth century, turned its focus to international tropical health issues. It was a Rockefeller-sponsored researcher, Hideyo Noguchi, who in the early 1920s confused the causative agent in leptospirosis with that of yellow fever, and created a vaccine to combat the newly identified culprit. By the early 1930s Noguchi's organism was out of favor, and he himself had died of yellow fever. Rockefeller researchers returned to the filterable virus first recognized by the Reed Commission in 1902, and, in 1936, Max Theiler created the first effective yellow fever vaccine. During that same decade scientists discovered the jungle cycle of yellow fever, which did not require the presence of humans for its continuation. With that discovery came the realization that although yellow fever might be severely limited in the human population through vaccine administration, it was an unlikely candidate for eradication.[20]

During World War II, U.S. public health officials were newly concerned with the possible importation of yellow fever. In the reports of the Malaria Control for War Areas agency (the Centers for Disease Control prototype), malaria was the principal concern, but yellow fever and typhus also received attention. The writer of the 1943 *Report* glued a toy airplane to a child's globe and photographed it to make the point that yellow fever mosquitoes and those infected could be rapidly conveyed by this increasingly prevalent mode of transportation. In response, public health officials sprayed planes before landing to kill any possible mosquitoes, and questioned those on board for symptoms of yellow fever. Apparently, there were no imported cases.[21]

During the 1950s Fred Soper and others who worked with the Rockefeller Foundation and the Pan American Health Organization called for the eradication of the *Aedes aegypti* mosquito from the western hemisphere. Soper had become famous for his feat of terminating the *Anopheles gambiae* malaria vector in Brazil, after its importation from Africa in the 1930s. He saw no reason, especially given the new powerful tool of DDT, that *aedes* species should not follow their African cousin into hemispheric extinction. With Rockefeller money, Soper's followers made a major dent in the numbers of *aedes* mosquitoes in Central and South America. U.S. officials were less enthusiastic and cooperative, and while the *aedes* population was diminished, eradication was never achieved. The *aedes* population has gradually resurged, and there is a new yellow fever vector in the American South now, *Aedes albopictus*. However, at least at present, yellow fever is no longer a significant public health issue in North America.[22]

HISTORIANS AND YELLOW FEVER

This sketch of yellow fever in the United States serves as the backdrop for a broader consideration of the historiography of yellow fever and public health. Yellow fever has attracted historical scrutiny for a variety of reasons. On the most basic level, the story of yellow fever epidemics makes good copy. A number of studies have recounted the drama in different locales, following in essence the same saga. The first cases appear; physicians and government officials try to hush it up; the disease spreads inexorably; people flee in panic; too little is done too late; hundreds or thousands die; isolated instances of heroism are identified. Such descriptive accounts fill the basic need of identifying when and where epidemics occurred, and often of outlining contemporary viewpoints on the disease. The studies of Louisiana by Duffy, Carrigan, and Gillson; of Memphis by Ellis and Baker; of the Mississippi Valley in 1878 by Bloom, and on Tallahassee by Miller all fall into this category.[23] However, in recent historiography this kind of descriptive work appears largely in medical journals with an interest in local history, such as recent accounts of Port Royal, South Carolina in the *Journal of the South Carolina Medical Association*, or of Norfolk, Virginia in the *Virginia Medical Quarterly*.[24]

Other historians have been interested in trying to apply current knowledge to past epidemics in an attempt to sort out "what really happened." They seek to elucidate what environmental, social, epidemiological, or economic factors favored the appearance and spread of yellow fever. Their work is similar to those who seek to make retrospective diagnoses of historical figures, and at least as fraught with difficulty. The earliest and most exhaustive of this genre is Henry Rose Carter's discussion of whether yellow fever origi-

189

nated in Africa or South America (akin to similar debates about syphilis and Columbus).[25] On a less global scale, David Geggus has analyzed the yellow fever epidemics in Santo Domingo in the 1790s with the ambition of understanding the severity and mortality of those especially epidemic years in the Caribbean. He finds his answers in the societal havoc of war, excessive movement of people from one island to another, and the presence of large numbers of susceptible British troops.[26] Smith and Gibson have looked at the now famous epidemic in South Wales in 1865 and tracked the actual course of the epidemic from historical documents. They credit the unusually mild summer and fortuitous shipboard events for the one and only appearance in Wales of yellow fever.[27] The most ambitious of such papers is James Goodyear's study of yellow fever and its relation to the sugar trade. He argues persuasively that an important factor in the nurturance and travel patterns of the yellow fever mosquito was the paraphernalia of sugar syrup refining and transport.[28]

Other historians have taken as their principal concern the process by which yellow fever changed epidemiological and etiological knowledge. The best of these is undeniably William Coleman's book comparing the response to epidemics in Saint-Nazaire, France (1861) and Swansea, Wales (1865). His principal focus is on the research of François Mélier and George Buchanan, who explored the epidemics in their respective countries. Mélier, especially, brought new precision to epidemiology, tracking in detail each new case and confirming with solid evidence the course of the fever through the port city of Saint-Nazaire. Both he and Buchanan came to the conclusion that the disease had been imported into their communities.[29]

Coleman recognizes the unique set of circumstances that allowed these two men to reach what at the time was a startling conclusion. "In northern Europe yellow fever had acted within a natural laboratory," he notes. "In effect it generated there a set of natural experiments. Unlike tropical ports, northern shores provided a yellow-fever-free background against which all parameters could be tested." Coleman's heroes were men in the right place at the right time. They escaped from the limited either-or thinking which had led the contagionist-anticontagionist battles to a draw by deciding to study the motion of the disease while admitting ignorance of its cause. Theirs was an epidemiology without an etiology. As a result, they demonstrated conclusively by means of careful figures and mapping that yellow fever had spread from infected ships through their towns.[30]

Mélier approached his task from an undeniably practical perspective. He was not all that interested in establishing the identity of yellow fever's etiological agent. Prevention was his main object, and to that end his careful report supported the reinstitution of limited quarantine in France. Coleman compares this outcome to the British case, where the Swansea experience was less persuasive. In part he finds that this was due to national styles in public policy; he also credits the unsympathetic attitude of Buchanan's superior, John Simon, to the lack of influence of the Welsh findings.[31] Two other studies have found nearly identical epidemiological conclusions being drawn in locales far distant from Coleman's epidemic sites. K. David Patterson has explored an epidemic in the Cape Verde Islands that occurred in 1846, and I have looked at the development of transportability theory in the American South in the 1840s.[32] What is interesting is the independence of the thinkers from each other. The physicians I studied wrote before Mélier and Buchanan, but were not known to the latter physicians. The report of the Cape Verde epidemic was mentioned in works that Mélier or Buchanan may have known, but was not particularly influential. The wheel was rediscovered several times. Coleman and I came to our conclusions independently as well, with both of us focusing on the small town with rare yellow fever as the best locus for recognizing yellow fever's portability.

One can postulate the confluence of a number of factors to explain the emergence of the transportability viewpoint at multiple loci. It was becoming more common at the time for physicians to believe yellow fever was a specific disease, and perhaps that its cause was accordingly specific, even if present in amorphous filth. The disease's resurgence at mid-century also coincided with nascent public health movements both in Europe and the United States. It directly challenged the authority of these newly established guardians of the public health. Yellow fever was a disease that could not be ignored, yet was devilishly difficult to explain. This tension generated an energy for research and action rarely spawned by more endemic diseases.

Issues of scientific priority have also spurred historians of yellow fever. For no aspect of its history is this more marked than the question of the discovery of the yellow fever vector. Josiah Clark Nott of Mobile is credited with being the first to mention, in 1848, mosquitoes in the etiology of yellow fever, but his concept was not that of the modern mosquito vector, and his writings now earn him no more than a footnote.[33] However, the storm continues to swirl around the figure of Carlos Finlay, a Cuban physician who published his suspicions about the mosquito and yellow fever before Walter Reed, although he did not succeed in convincing the world as Reed's famous experiments did. There is much debate about whether Reed actually depended on Finlay's work, or, alternatively, if the discoveries about the malaria vector made by Ronald Ross and Giovanni Grassi in the years 1897 and 1898 were more directly influential. François Delaporte takes on the origins of Reed's ideas, a major case study on the question of scientific creativity, and both thoroughly airs the Finlay enthusiasts' claims and attributes key status to a group of visiting physicians from Liverpool. Nationality obviously plays a part, with almost all works about Finlay appearing in Spanish, while Reed is an American national hero with an eponymous major U.S. army hospital. Although the account of the issue of priority occupied only a few pages in my book on yellow fever, its reviewer in the *New England Journal of Medicine* felt called upon to devote over half of his review to this discussion, in order to "set the record straight." The conversations about Reed and Finlay are quite similar to those about the first use of anesthesia; determining priority, not the time of acceptance and widespread use, becomes the rather short-sighted goal.[34]

REFLECTIONS AND SPECULATIONS

For the nineteenth century one can argue that yellow fever was the disease that inspired the most permanent public health reform in America. "While the quarantinable diseases as defined by our regulations are nominally cholera, smallpox, yellow fever, typhus fever, plague and leprosy," summed up one federal public health official in 1897, "still it is only yellow fever whose shadow ever crosses our path, and is always a source of dread, a constant source of expense, and at once a danger to our people and an onerous burden upon commerce."[35] Certainly yellow fever was central to the origins of federal public health involvement, and it had a vast impact on southern state boards of health as well. Its very elusiveness made it the center of debates about public health theory and practice, eliciting progression in the sophistication of epidemiological techniques. The history of yellow fever provides a useful model for understanding the ways in which one disease can provoke research and reform that have far-reaching implications for science and society.

An interesting pattern does emerge from the yellow fever experience that is more broadly applicable to the history of public health. When physicians were divided over quarantine versus sanitation, and the efficacy of neither appeared clear cut, politicians were reluctant to fund large public health projects. Reform in any direction was stunted, and failed efforts at street cleaning or isolation hailed loudly by those protecting the taxpayer's pocketbook from wasteful expenditures. Only when the disease was on the doorstep did politicians vote feeble funds to bar the door. This changed in the 1880s. The concept of disinfection offered the possibility of a truly protective quarantine that was at the same time limited and relatively cheap. Businessmen compared the alternatives between commerce-disrupting epidemics and disinfecting quarantine stations, and chose the latter. Here was a technique that anyone could understand: acid gas would kill disease-causing germs and purify the ship or train, allowing it to continue on its journey in a few days. The city was safe; the cargo was safe. Funds for such quarantine stations repeatedly appeared in state and federal budgets in the 1880s and 1890s. They probably did a fair job of killing mosquitoes, which accounts for their good record of success.[36]

The yellow fever experience would suggest that in order to gain political support in the United States a public health measure had best meet the following criteria: (1) be grounded in undisputed medical theory; (2) be reasonably inexpensive; (3) afford minimal disruption of individual rights; (4) target a public health menace which threatens a significant portion of the population; and (5) have a mode of action that is fairly straightforward and comprehensible to the lay mind. By the latter I mean that cause and effect are direct and easy to visualize. By the 1880s the etiology of yellow fever, at least at the level of "germ causes disease," was disputed only by the cranky few. The identity of the germ was eagerly sought, but no leading physician doubted its existence or that it would succumb to the disinfecting powers of chloride and sulphur as other germs did. The disinfecting station was expensive to establish, but less so than the cost of one epidemic, and certainly less than the old-fashioned "forty days in isolation" quarantines. While the scientific quarantine did interfere with the free movement of people and things, the loss of liberty was not felt too burdensome. Further, yellow fever was a dreadful disease that clearly required prevention. Finally, the technique had clear analogies for the lay mind to latch onto. The disinfecting stations killed germs just as the army would kill invading soldiers. The combination was right for generating government action in public health.[37]

So, is yellow fever "done" or are there new directions for research? The essays in this volume suggest that new research strategies have much to offer beyond 1793. The dissection of "communities" of yellow fever response offers a particularly promising mode for analyzing cities and towns struck with yellow fever. Consideration of medical and other public writings on the disease as genres is equally intriguing. Certainly the anonymous pre-publication reviewer of my book who pointed to the dearth of attention to race in its pages was spot on. Yellow fever was largely a southern disease, and the South was defined for the most part by its race relations. Beginnings have been made, such as Roussey's discussion of black policemen in Memphis in 1878–79, or my brief mention of the transformation of blacks from being considered at low risk for yellow fever to being seen as dangerous carriers. But more is needed, especially on the delicate question of variations of racial susceptibility to the disease, begun so thoughtfully by Kiple and King.[38]

Broader still are approaches suggested from outside the yellow fever historiography. To date, yellow fever studies have largely been locality-bound. Few historians have considered it in light of the "Atlantic System" in which it circulated. Southern ports shared the microorganisms of Cuba, Vera Cruz, and Rio de Janeiro because their ships and people traveled frequently to and from these localities. Considering yellow fever in New Orleans or Charleston without considering these cities as part of a broader community with the Caribbean, Central and South America, and the west coast of Africa misses the major network of epidemiological vectors that traversed the Atlantic. In some ways it makes more sense to see southern ports as part of the Caribbean community than as cities "in" the United States, especially in the era when sailing ships, and not trains or trucks, carried the bulk of commercial trade. Only the work of Philip Curtin has begun to chart the epidemiological pattern of this redefined "community."[39]

Further insights will come from studies of medical imperialism and international health. Certainly the growing bibliography of works on the role of the Rockefeller Foundation in Spanish America, Africa, and Asia reveals the power of this approach. First, the foundation was central to sponsoring laboratory research on the yellow fever virus, so its priorities in distributing such money become central to the yellow fever story.[40] From a more social history point of view, studies such as Armando Solorzano's essay on the Rockefeller Foundation's place in the conquest of yellow fever in Mexico raise interesting questions about the goals of third world public health.[41] In many ways the American South of the 1910s and 1920s was a "third world country"—its economic infrastructure was weak, its people the most impoverished in the country, educational and medical resources were primitive, and a large body of the people subsisted as agricultural peasants. Using analyses of the Rockefeller Foundation's pattern of action in Mexico or South America may provide intriguing insights into the Foundation's, and the U. S. Government's, approach to public health issues in the American South. To a certain extent it may be true that both entities "practiced" public health reform in their native "developing country" before taking on international health projects.

Some of the most fruitful insights for the history of public health have come from the field of medical anthropology. This is especially true of Mary Douglas's influential book *Purity and Danger*. This work describes the key place of purification rituals in keeping societies "safe," whether the impure item in question is a corpse, a menstruating woman, or a dollop of fecal material. Certainly, the history of yellow fever is enlightened by an awareness of such practices. The burning of tar in nineteenth-century streets to purify the air or the heating of blankets to 250 degrees to "kill the germ" are both examples of behaviors supported by societal constructs of purity. The quarantine itself, the forty days of ritual purgatory, is certainly tied to Judeo-Christian concepts of "purification periods." Beginning with the forty days of Noah and the forty years of Moses, the conceit is continued with Christ's forty days in the desert, and remembered with the forty days of Lent.[42] It is curious that the nineteenth-century United States, with its largely Protestant national religious ethic, apparently had forgotten the significance of the forty days. As quarantine's length was being debated in the South both before and after the Civil War, scientific evidence of surety had replaced any religious understanding as the basis for determining the period of detention. Further studies of the place of concepts of purity and purification in American public health history may yield equally interesting results.

Historians who wish to look again at yellow fever in the United States could take as their model no better work than that of Ken de Bevoise on epidemic disease in the Philippines around 1900.[43] This book, which analyzes a demographic crisis on multiple levels, including the health of cattle, the movement of peoples as determined by war and markets, the importation of disease, the role of malnutrition, and the bungling of imperial managers, sets a new standard for depth of investigation about the place of disease in society. The essays in this volume begin that intricate task for Philadelphia in 1793, but much remains to be done, especially around the complex issues of yellow fever's persistence in the American South. The new student of yellow fever should take heart—yes, there is still much to be done on this fascinating and horrible disease.

NOTES

1. Parts of this essay stem from a paper given at a symposium in memorial for William Coleman, "Epidemics and Their Social Impact," Madison, Wisconsin, 1989. My thanks to John Eyler and Judith Walzer Leavitt for their comments on this earlier paper, and to the editors of the current volume for their decision to include it along with the conference papers.

2. John Blake, "Yellow Fever in Eighteenth-Century America," *Bulletin of the New York Academy of Medicine* 44 (1968): 673–686; Jo Ann Carrigan, "Yellow Fever: Scourge of the South," in *Disease and Distinctiveness in the American South*, eds. Todd L. Savitt and James Harvey Young (Knoxville: University of Tennessee Press, 1988), pp. 55–78; K. David Patterson, "Yellow Fever Epidemics and Mortality in the United States, 1693–1905," *Social Science and Medicine* 34 (1992): 855–865.

3. Martin Pernick, "Politics, Parties, and Pestilence: Epidemic Yellow Fever in Philadelphia and the Rise of the First Party System," *William and Mary Quarterly*, 3rd. ser., 29 (1972): 559–586, and reprinted in this volume; J. H. Powell, *Bring Out Your Dead: The Great Plague of Yellow Fever in Philadelphia in 1793* (Philadelphia: University of Pennsylvania Press, 1949).

4. John Duffy, "Yellow Fever in the Continental United States during the Nineteenth Century," *Bulletin of the New York Academy of Medicine* 44 (1968): 687–701.

5. René La Roche, *Yellow Fever, Considered in Its Historical, Pathological, Etiological, and Therapeutic Relations* (Philadelphia: Blanchard and Son, 1855). Here and in much of what follows I condense material from my book, *Yellow Fever and the South* (New Brunswick: Rutgers University Press, 1992).

6. Margaret Warner [Humphreys], "Public Health in the Old South," in *Science and Medicine in the Old South*, eds. Ronald L. Numbers and Todd L. Savitt (Baton Rouge: Louisiana State University Press, 1989), pp. 226–255.

7. Margaret Warner [Humphreys], "Hunting the Yellow Fever Germ: The Principle

and Practice of Etiological Proof in Late Nineteenth Century America," *Bulletin of the History of Medicine* 59 (1985): 361–82; and William Bulloch, *The History of Bacteriology* (London: Oxford University Press, 1938).

8. Humphreys, *Yellow Fever and the South*; and J. C. Faget, "Type and Specific Character of True Yellow Fever, As Shown by Observations Taken with the Assistance of the Thermometer and Second-Hand Watch," *New Orleans Medical and Surgical Journal* 1 (1873–74): 145–168.

9. John Duffy, *The Sword of Pestilence: The New Orleans Yellow Fever Endemic of 1853* (Baton Rouge: Louisiana State University Press, 1966); and Gordon E. Gillson, *Louisiana State Board of Health: The Formative Years* (M.A. thesis, Lousiana State University and Agricultural and Mechanical College, 1967).

10. Stanford E. Chaillé, "The Yellow Fever, Sanitary Condition, and Vital Statistics of New Orleans during Its Military Occupation; The Four Years 1862–65," *New Orleans Journal of Medicine* 23 (1870): 563–598. George Augustin provided a list of outbreaks of yellow fever in the United States from 1860 to 1905 in *History of Yellow Fever* (New Orleans: Searcy and Pfaff, 1909), pp. 179–80.

11. Emory Q. Hawk, *Economic History of the South* (New York: Prentice Hall, 1934); J. Carlyle Sitterson, *Sugar Country: The Cane Sugar Industry in the South, 1753–1950* (Lexington: University of Kentucky Press, 1953); and John F. Stover, *The Railroads of the South, 1865–1900: A Study in Finance and Control* (Chapel Hill: University of North Carolina Press, 1955).

12. Margaret Warner [Humphreys], "Local Control Versus National Interest: The Debate over Southern Public Health, 1878–1884," *Journal of Southern History* 50 (1984): 407–28. The statistics are from J. M. Woodworth, "A Brief Review of the Organization and Purpose of the Yellow Fever Commission," *Reports and Papers of the American Public Health Association* 4 (1877–78): 167–168.

13. Humphreys, *Yellow Fever and the South*.

14. One of the best and most detailed accounts of the employment of germicidal techniques against yellow fever is George M. Sternberg et al., *Disinfection and Disinfectants: Their Application and Use in the Prevention and Treatment of Disease, and in Public and Private Sanitation* (Concord, N.H.: Republican Press Association for the American Public Health Association, 1888).

15. Peter Bruton, "The National Board of Health" (Ph.D. diss., University of Maryland, 1974).

16. Humphreys, *Yellow Fever and the South*; and Ralph Chester Williams, *The United States Public Health Service, 1798–1950* (Washington: Commissioned Officers Association of the USPHS, 1951).

17. Howard A. Kelly, *Walter Reed and Yellow Fever* (New York: McClure, Phillips and Co., 1906); and William B. Bean, *Walter Reed: A Biography* (Charlottesville: University Press of Virginia, 1982).

18. Marie D. Gorgas and Burton S. Hendrick, *William Crawford Gorgas: His Life and Work* (Philadelphia: Lea and Febiger, 1924).

19. Humphreys, *Yellow Fever and the South*, chapter 5.

20. Wilbur G. Downs, "History of Epidemiological Aspects of Yellow Fever," *Yale Journal of Biology and Medicine* 55 (1982): 179–185; George K. Strode, ed., *Yellow*

Fever (New York: McGraw-Hill Book Co., 1951); and John Z. Bowers and Edith E. King, "The Conquest of Yellow Fever: The Rockefeller Foundation," *Journal of the Medical Society of New Jersey* 78 (1981): 539–541.

21. *Malaria Control in War Areas Reports*, 1941–45. See also Margaret Humphreys, "Kicking a Dying Dog: DDT and the Demise of Malaria in the American South, 1942–1950," *Isis* 87 (1996): 1–17.

22. Thomas P. Monath, "Yellow Fever: *Victor, Victoria?* Conqueror, Conquest? Epidemics and Research in the Last Forty Years and Prospects for the Future," *American Journal of Tropical Medicine* 45 (1991): 1–43.

23. Duffy, *Sword of Pestilence*; Gillson, *Louisiana State Board of Health*; Jo Ann Carrigan, *The Saffron Scourge: A History of Yellow Fever in Louisiana. 1796–1905* (Lafayette, La.: Center for Louisiana Studies, 1994); Thomas H. Baker, "Yellowjack: The Yellow Fever Epidemic of 1878 in Memphis, Tennessee," *Bulletin of the History of Medicine* 42 (1968): 241–264; John H. Ellis, *Yellow Fever and Public Health in the New South* (Lexington: The University Press of Kentucky, 1992); Khaled J. Bloom, *The Mississippi Valley's Great Yellow Fever Epidemic of 1878* (Baton Rouge: Louisiana State University Press, 1993); and Barbara Elizabeth Miller, "Tallahassee and the 1841 Yellow Fever Epidemic" (M.A. thesis, Florida State University, 1976).

24. See Elizabeth Young Newsom, "South Carolina's Last Yellow Fever Epidemic: Manning Simons at Port Royal, 1877," *Journal of the South Carolina Medical Association* 7 (1995): 311–313; and Penelope Barlow Lewis and Donald W. Lewis, "Deathstorm: The Yellow Fever Epidemic of 1855," *Virginia Medical Quarterly* 122 (1995): 38–42.

25. Henry Rose Carter, *Yellow Fever: An Historical and Epidemiological Study of Its Place of Origin* (Baltimore: Williams & Wilkins, 1931).

26. David Geggus. "Yellow Fever in the 1790s: The British Army in Occupied Saint Domingue," *Medical History* 23 (1979): 38–58.

27. C. E. Gordon Smith and Mary E. Gibson, "Yellow Fever in South Wales, 1865," *Medical History* 30 (1986): 322–340.

28. James D. Goodyear, "The Sugar Connection: A New Perspective on the History of Yellow Fever," *Bulletin of the History of Medicine* 52 (1978): 5–21.

29. William Coleman, *Yellow Fever in the North: The Methods of Early Epidemiology* (Madison: University of Wisconsin Press, 1987).

30. The quotation is from Coleman's first publication concerning this material, "Epidemiological Method in the 1860s: Yellow Fever at Saint-Nazaire," *Bulletin of the History of Medicine* 58 (1984): 145–163, quote on p. 162.

31. Coleman, *Yellow Fever in the North*.

32. K. David Patterson, "Epidemiology in the Mid-Nineteenth Century: The Case of the 1845–46 Yellow Fever Epidemic at Boa Vista," in *History of Epidemiology*, eds. Yosio Kawakita et al. (Tokyo: Japan Printing Co., Ltd., 1993), pp. 59–91; Warner [Humphreys], "Public Health in the Old South."

33. Reginald Horsman, *Josiah Nott of Mobile* (Baton Rouge: Louisiana State University Press, 1987); and Eli Chernin, "Josiah Clark Nott, Insects, and Yellow Fever," *Bulletin of the New York Academy of Medicine* 59 (1983): 790–802.

34. François Delaporte, *The History of Yellow Fever: An Essay on the Birth of Tropical*

Fever, trans. Arthur Goldhammer (Cambridge: The MIT Press, 1991; first French ed. 1989); Juan A. del Regato, "Carlos Finlay and the Nobel Prize in Physiology or Medicine," *The Pharos* (Spring, 1987): 5–9; R. D. Rumbaut, "Review of *Yellow Fever and the South*," *New England Journal of Medicine* 328 (1993): 1793–1795.

35. H. D. Geddings, "Yellow Fever from a Clinical and Epidemiological Point of View and Its Relation to the Quarantine System of the United States," *Report of the Marine Hospital Service* (1897), p. 241.

36. Humphreys, *Yellow Fever and the South*.

37. Ibid.

38. Dennis C. Rousey, "Yellow Fever and Black Policemen in Memphis: A Post-Reconstruction Anomaly," *Journal of Southern History* 51 (1985): 357–74; Humphreys, *Yellow Fever and the South*, pp. 164–65; Kenneth Kiple and Virginia King, "Black Yellow Fever Immunities, Both Acquired and Innate as Revealed in the American South," *Social Science History* 1 (1977): 419–36. See also Susan E. Klepp's essay in this volume.

39. Philip Curtin, "Epidemiology and the Slave Trade," *Political Science Quarterly* 83 (1967): 190–216; idem, *Death by Migration: Europe's Encounter with the Tropical World in the Nineteenth Century* (Cambridge: Cambridge University Press, 1989). My conception of the Atlantic Rim has benefited from conversations with Janet Ewald and David Barry Gaspar.

40. Bowers and King, "The Conquest of Yellow Fever."

41. Armando Solorzano, "Sowing the Seeds of Neo-Imperialism: The Rockefeller Foundation's Yellow Fever Campaign in Mexico," *International Journal of Health Services* 22 (1992): 529–554; see also Marcos Cueto, ed., *Missionaries of Science: The Rockefeller Foundation and Latin America* (Bloomington: Indiana University Press, 1994).

42. Genesis 7.4; Exodus 16.35; Mark 1.12.

43. Ken de Bevoise, *Agents of the Apocalypse: Epidemic Disease in the Colonial Philippines* (Princeton: Princeton University Press, 1995).

Notes on Contributors

J. WORTH ESTES, M.D. is Professor of Pharmacology at the Boston University School of Medicine. His research specialty is the therapeutic practices of the eighteenth and nineteenth centuries. The author or co-editor of many works on various aspects of the history of medicine, his most recent books are the *Dictionary of Protopharmacology: Therapeutic Practices, 1700–1850* (Science History Publications, 1990) and *Naval Surgeon: Life and Death at Sea in the Age of Sail* (Science History Publications, 1997). He is the Secretary-Treasurer of the American Association for the History of Medicine and Editor of the *Journal of the History of Medicine and Allied Sciences.*

SALLY F. GRIFFITH, Ph.D. is an independent scholar who has taught American history at Villanova University. The author of *Home Town News: William Allen White and the Emporia Gazette,* she is currently completing *Public-Spirited Enterprise,* a study on boosterism in America from Benjamin Franklin to the present. She is also researching a history of the Historical Society of Pennsylvania during the past seventy-five years.

MARGARET HUMPHREYS, M.D., Ph.D. teaches history and practices medicine at Duke University. She is the author of *Yellow Fever and the South* (Rutgers University Press, 1992) and is currently at work on a history of malaria in the United States.

SUSAN E. KLEPP, Ph.D. is Professor of History at Rider University. Among her books are *Philadelphia in Transition: A Demographic History of the City and Its Occupational Groups, 1720–1830* (American Philosophical Society, 1989); *"The Swift Progress of Population": A Documentary and Bibliographic Study of Philadelphia's Growth* (American Philosophical Society, 1991); and *The Infortunate: The Voyage and Adventure of William Moraley, an Indentured Servant* [with Billy G. Smith] (Penn State University Press, 1992).

PHILLIP LAPSANSKY is Chief of Reference at the Library Company of Philadelphia and curator of the library's Afro-Americana Collection. His current research is on American racial graphics, and he is compiling a selection of books and pamphlets from the collection for microform republication.

MICHAL MCMAHON, Ph.D. is Associate Professor of History at West Virginia University, where he specializes in eighteenth- and nineteenth-century American and environmental history. He is currently writing a history of the formation of early Philadelphia.

JACQUELYN C. MILLER, Ph.D. is Assistant Professor of History at Seattle University. She is co-editor of *Benjamin Rush, M.D.: A Bibliographic Guide* (Greenwood Press, 1996), and is currently editing a book on the formation of class identities in eighteenth-century America.

DAVID PAUL NORD, Ph.D. is Professor of Journalism and American Studies and Adjunct Professor of History at Indiana University, Bloomington. His current research interests lie in the history of religious publishing and the history of reading and readers. He is former Associate Editor and Acting Editor of the *Journal of American History*.

MARTIN S. PERNICK, Ph.D. is Professor of History at the University of Michigan. His research interests include the history of ethical issues in medicine and the role of medicine in mass culture. He has taught at Harvard University and at Penn State University's Hershey Medical Center. He is the author of *A Calculus of Suffering* (Columbia University Press, 1985) and *The Black Stork: Eugenics and the Death of "Defective" Babies in American Medicine and Motion Pictures Since 1915* (Oxford University Press, 1996).

BILLY G. SMITH, Ph.D. is Professor of History at Montana State University. Among his publications are *The "Lower Sort": Philadelphia's Laboring People, 1750–1800* (Cornell University Press, 1990); *The Infortunate: The Voyage and Adventure of William Moraley, an Indentured Servant* [with Susan E. Klepp] (Penn State University Press, 1992); *Blacks Who Stole Themselves: Advertisements for Runaways in the Pennsylvania Gazette, 1728–1790* [with Richard Wojtowicz] (University of Pennsylvania Press, 1989); *Life in Early Philadelphia: Documents from the Revolutionary and Early National Periods* (Penn State University Press, 1995). Currently he is completing a book about runaway slaves in eighteenth-century America.

Index

Numbers in italics indicate illustrations; numbers followed by "n" indicate notes; numbers followed by "t" indicate tables.

THE COLLEGE OF PHYSICIANS OF PHILADELPHIA, founded in 1787 by 24 of the city's leading physicians, including Benjamin Rush, a signer of the Declaration of Independence, and John Morgan, founder of America's first medical school, is a not-for-profit educational and cultural institution dedicated to promoting a greater understanding of medicine and the roles of the physician in contemporary society. The College carries out its mission through its various programs, including its Library, C. Everett Koop Community Health Information Center, Mutter Museum, and Francis Clark Wood Institute for the History of Medicine. Since its founding, the College has been actively involved in community service, particularly in the area of public health. The College's fellowship (as its approximately 2,000 elected members are known collectively) is comprised of many nationally recognized leaders of America's health care profession.

THE LIBRARY COMPANY OF PHILADELPHIA is an independent research library which preserves over half a million rare books, prints, and photographs documenting every aspect of American history and culture from the 17th through the 19th centuries. It is a research center serving a national and international constituency of scholars. The Library Company was founded in 1731 by Benjamin Franklin as a subscription library supported by shareholders, as it is to this day. The Library Company is open to the public free of charge, and carries out its mission by maintaining reading rooms, increasing and cataloguing the collections, mounting exhibitions, producing publications for both scholarly and general audiences, offering research grants and fellowships to graduate students and senior scholars, and presenting public programs.